The Diet Doc
Metabolic Manual

Joe Klemczewski, Ph.D.

To order additional copies of this book, contact:
A3R Labs, Inc., dba The Diet Doc
812-868-8710
8601 N. Kentucky Ave., Suite G
Evansville, IN 47725

TABLE OF CONTENTS

Chapter One

GETTING STARTED

Congratulations! You've made the decision to become your own nutritionist and that is the biggest step you'll take in making weight loss permanent! The book you're holding is a no-fluff, nuts-and-bolts version of my Metabolic Transformation program developed over the span of a decade. Thousands of people have achieved weight-loss goals and gained control for life using the information you're about to read. Be patient, though, I'm asking you to be my partner in the process.

There are two reasons people fail on diets and end up gaining weight back. The first is structural. I emphasize the science and physiology of nutrition and weight loss because I know it's critical for long-term success. Simple but numerous illustrations will help you understand your body so you don't have to be a slave to dieting over and over and over… I do want you to become your own nutritionist, but just like learning a new skill, a new language, or a musical instrument, it will take digging your heels in and committing to a learning process. I think you can achieve you the body you want, save years of frustrating dieting, and may even save your life. Many diets simply aren't safe or can leave your metabolism suppressed, setting you up for fast regain. The structure of your diet has to be one that works with your body, not against it.

The second reason diets fail is that they're too rigid. You're asked to eliminate major food groups, choose meals from a limited exchange list, or do horribly impractical things. I know it can be easy initially to just have someone tell you exactly what, when, and how much to eat, but in the long run you will fail. Learning to be flexible and how to thrive in any circumstance you find yourself is the only way you can make a diet successful long-term. Trust me when I say the payoff is actually enjoying that flexibility forever. Imagine being able to eat some "bad" foods while you diet and still lose. Imagine never regaining weight back. Compare that to doing something unnatural all the way through a diet and then you're asked to eat "normally" again without gaining weight back. What's "normal?" Normal to me is learning to eat the foods you like, achieving your goals now, and winning permanently. It's not eating tree bark and bird seed or starving yourself. It's building meal patterns into your day that you like and that work. Normal is you and I working together to merge the nutrition knowledge necessary with YOUR life and making progress.

I've got a big head start on our partnership by dumping my life's work into these pages. While you'll learn there are many ways of applying it due to our uniqueness, this text will create a foundation that you can build on endlessly. There's nothing worse than climbing a ladder for a long time and finding it was up against the wrong wall. You're now on the right ladder on the right wall. For your part, you're going to need some tools. Don't let this scare you, but I'd get a digital food scale ($30.00 will buy a nice one), a food count book (I'm a big fan of *The Complete Book of Food Counts* by Corrine Netzer), and a calculator. That's it. Me: *Metabolic Manual*, you: a little math. Partners.

That gives us some work to do, so buckle up. But first, my friend and writing partner on an expanded version of this book, Dr. Scott Uloth, M.D., wouldn't be happy if I let you get started without reminding you to see your doctor to make sure your health is stable and safe enough to participate in a weight-loss program. He's right. So hurry up, I'm ready to get started!

CHAPTER ONE KEY POINTS

▸ 1) Metabolic Transformation is based on solid science.

▸ 2) Be can active participant in your success.

▸ 3) No one is the same metabolically or personally. While providing the right structure, Metabolic Transformation allows maximum flexibility.

▸ 4) See your physician for a physical – you're overdue.

▸ 5) Take responsibility, be consistent, track your food, learn, and permanent success will be yours.

Chapter Two

THE DIET DOC Rx

Metabolism Defined

Not long ago, a 44-year-old man came to me with a goal of getting leaner and possibly gaining some muscle. He already enjoyed a lifestyle of working out and running almost every day and had done so for most of his adult life. Despite being very healthy from his physical training perspective, he gained and lost 20 pounds more than once and like many of us, despised his lack of control. He wanted to lose weight again, but he also wanted a permanent change and permanent control. His experience begs the question of whether people need more motivation and effort or if the design of a particular diet may be flawed. Are we failing because we're not disciplined or is the diet failing us? There is an intertwining of the physiological and the psychological aspects of weight loss that cannot be separated. A great number of failed dieters feel tremendous guilt about not being disciplined when it may be simply that they don't understand the physiology of what's happening and what they can do to positively affect it. I can't tell you how many times I've heard, "I have control over every aspect of my life except my weight. Why?!" The physical and mental sides of diet affect each other in a very dynamic relationship. As you'll learn in the rest of this chapter, the first week of changing your nutrition brings about significant changes within your body, literally creating stability that makes it easier than you think to not only lose weight, but to do it without suffering. "Attainable and sustainable" is the phrase you can use to describe *Metabolic Transformation.*

My new client lost 20 pounds of body fat and gained 5 pounds of lean muscle mass in his first 8 weeks. How can a man who already exercises regularly, works out with weights at least four days per week, and runs in road races have such dramatic results just by changing his nutrition? The answer is metabolism. He actually complained of having to eat so much food on his program, yet after these first eight weeks I had to increase his food so he wouldn't lose weight "too quickly." He often commented on his new, higher level of energy. A very disciplined, in-control person, he went as far as saying, "Coming to you literally changed my life." Are these the typical comments of dieters you know? Study after study has shown most dieters regain even more weight than they lose on any given plan. It need not be. We're going for permanent results, not just a temporary fix.

How many times have you heard people say they have a fast or slow metabolism? Thin people often say, "I have a fast metabolism," and those who are overweight often say, "I have a slow metabolism." We are quick to blame or credit our body size on a word that most of us don't understand. Basal metabolic rate is the rate at which your body burns calories over a specific amount of time. It's true that there is some variability in everyone's metabolism; however, I have met few people who had a legitimately "slow" metabolism due to a thyroid imbalance, metabolic condition, or medical ailment that would compromise weight loss. In other words, your metabolism may be slightly lower than someone else's, but it is probably not the reason you are overweight.

The cause of your weight struggle likely goes beyond your genetic metabolism; though for a small percentage of people, genetics do play a major role in making it easier to gain weight. Hormone levels that were immeasurable just years ago are being found to be major players in weight loss and gain. These hormones directly control metabolism, fat storage, and even hunger levels. The number of genetic fat cells can even be significantly different between people making it harder for some to lose weight. There is great research being done on morbid obesity that will help a lot of people, but most of us are overweight by our own eating habits.

Don't misunderstand me. While I'm downplaying the role of metabolism as an excuse, it does play a great role with long-term impact in the big picture of weight management. What you eat does affect your metabolism. Within weeks, you can raise or lower your body's ability to burn calories, sometimes significantly. Over time, this change can add up to large weight loss or gain. To be quite honest, this is the foundation of permanent weight loss. By eating the right amount of food, eating within the right daily structure, consuming better ratios of the three macronutrients (protein, carbohydrates, and fat), selecting the right food choices, and learning to be consistent, you can actually increase the amount of calories your body burns per day. This change in metabolism is due to the optimum operation of your body's internal environment.

(Figure 2:1) Basal Metabolic Rate

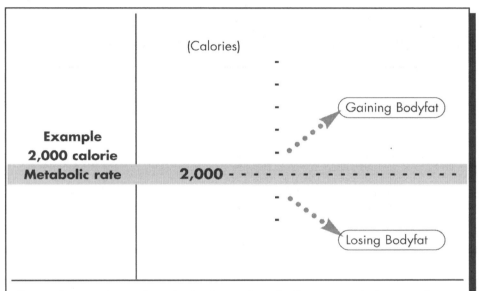

Eating fewer calories than the body needs is the first step to losing weight, however, done improperly will cause the body to decrease calorie burning making it easier to gain body fat. Permanent, positive changes in metabolism will occur only through the combined results of eating nutrients in the right amounts in a structured meal plan.

When you diet or eat incorrectly, your body does not work at optimum levels. Know anyone who has lost 30 pounds only to gain 40 back? They may insist they didn't gorge themselves to regain the weight but simply started eating "normally." Incorrect dieting can reduce the amount of calories your body burns, therefore making it much easier to gain weight even though you're trying to lose weight. Pay close attention to the details of this book as we explore how your body works with correct eating and diet.

AVERAGE JOE PHYSIOLOGY

The Straight Scoop on Metabolism

Numerous studies show how quickly our bodies can be affected by changes in diet. The dreaded "slow metabolism" isn't to be blamed by most of us; the super-sized lunches, chips, snacks, double helpings at dinner, and the worn track from the couch to the kitchen are the real culprits. But when we chose to embark on a weight-loss plan, we can do some short-term damage to our metabolism by incorrect eating.

A study showed that after 24 days of low-calorie dieting (450 calories – that's low!) the metabolism can be decreased by 15%. Several studies have reported decreases in resting metabolic rate up to 20 to 30%. Dropping your metabolism that fast means you're likely to regain more weight back when you start "eating normally" again until your metabolism catches back up, which it will do. In extreme cases, such as anorexia, metabolic rates have been measured to be slashed by 45%.

You may not be aware that just as eating too little decreases your metabolic rate, overeating increases it. This is where we lose the "I'm fat because of a slow metabolism" excuse. One study showed that when subjects who required 3,100 calories to maintain their weight gained 20% or more of their initial weight, they had to eat 5,100 calories to maintain that extra weight due to a heightened metabolism. (That gives credence to some who say, "I don't eat enough, that's why I can't lose weight." The metabolism is very sensitive and needs to sometimes be "rebuilt," but changes have to be made incrementally.

The importance of small changes is shown clearly in "yo-yo" dieting. Going on and off of diets repeatedly makes it more difficult to lose weight. Remember, the negative effects are short-term and your metabolism can be corrected, but the damage (weight regain) can be done so fast that you actually regain more weight than you lost. One study took subjects through two cycles of weight loss and weight regain. The rate of loss was only half during the second cycle compared to the first and the rate of regain was increased by 300%! That means when you diet and then binge and then diet again, you are only 50% as effective metabolically than the first round, and when your metabolism is suppressed from the dieting, you regain weight back 3 times faster than if you hadn't dieted at all. (That's how sensitive your metabolism is and why you need to have a knowledge base to guide you to successful and permanent weight loss. Scott got to experience this

continued ⟶

AVERAGE JOE PHYSIOLOGY

firsthand over the holidays when we first worked together. Already doing great with his weight loss, he thought, "Hey, I'm exercising, I'm doing great; I can eat all this sugar and fat and just burn it off." One dessert led to another, party after party, and 17 pounds later, reality set in. It took months to re-lose that weight and he learned that you can't outsmart your metabolism.

Eating the Right Amount to Raise Your Metabolism

As we progress through specific nutrient information and physiology, you will clearly see how the amount, type, and consumption pattern of food can literally accelerate your metabolism to full throttle. The first and most important step, however, is to estimate your metabolic rate correctly so you can eat the right amount of food that allows you to reach your weight-loss goals. Once you know how much energy your body requires, you can adjust your eating downward to begin the weight-loss process.

You could logically assume that eating 5 calories less than your body requires burns 5 extra calories stored as body fat, or that if you consume 500 calories less, your body makes up the difference by burning 500 calories of stored fat. Actually, the process is more complex than this. There is far more to permanent weight loss than just reducing calories. For instance, the body can burn calories by catabolizing, or breaking down, other tissues such as muscle. Even if your goals don't include gaining muscle, the last thing you want to do is lose lean body mass. Retaining muscle is too important for long-term metabolic function, strength, energy, and even in preventing osteoporosis. Other "intermediate" sources of energy such as blood sugar and stored carbohydrates (glycogen) in the liver and muscle may be used as well. Thus, the goal is to maximize fat loss while sparing muscle. There is a fine line between losing the most body fat as fast as possible and doing it in such a way that your metabolism is raised and not lowered.

The first step is to determine the right amount of food necessary to reach your goal. I have developed a chart based on gender and height to make this most important step very easy. This chart ensures enough food to avoid any deficiencies in the three macronutrients, and is geared towards a one-to-two pound weight loss per week. A great deal of experience and human trial has been

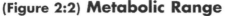

(Figure 2:2) Metabolic Range

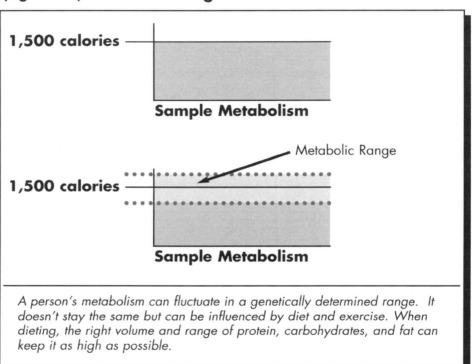

A person's metabolism can fluctuate in a genetically determined range. It doesn't stay the same but can be influenced by diet and exercise. When dieting, the right volume and range of protein, carbohydrates, and fat can keep it as high as possible.

poured into this chart to make it simple as well as the most powerful tool you have ever had in your battle for permanent weight control. It seems too easy to just plug yourself into a chart and follow the numbers, but therein lies the challenge. It will require discipline to stay with your program. Most people reading this will not have a clear concept regarding the numbers on the chart. In other words, most cannot correlate how much food is required to eat 100 grams of protein or even what foods contain protein. Don't worry; within six weeks you will be on the way to becoming your own nutritionist. Thousands of clients have found this plan to provide the most attainable and sustainable results ever experienced. A significant help is the flexibility you have in food selection yet the strict guidance you have in your personal macronutrient range profile. This chart is the cornerstone of the program. All of the science contained in the book is funneled into this tool, The Diet Doc Rx.

Those of you that want something simple; here it is. Eat within the levels appropriate for your gender and height and you'll lose weight. You and I both know, though, that it's more than just hitting a gram or calorie total. Knowing what to eat, how to structure your day nutritionally, plan meals, and learning about the individuality of your body is what pays dividends long after you set this book aside.

What if It Doesn't Seem to Be Working?

Everything we will explore from this point will define this one simple step of consuming the right amounts of the three macronutrients. I will expand and explain a great deal of information that will make this step even easier, yet it is still your responsibility to stay within the levels on this chart. It won't require weird foods (like pomegranate or grilled alligator) or crazy behaviors (like sit-ups hanging from your garage rafters or pushing a cart through snowy Russian mountains as in *Rocky IV*), just discipline. There are two very different definitions of the word discipline. The first is punishment. As soon as you read the word discipline related to weight loss, I know it sounds like punishment. However, the second definition is your definition: to train or develop by instruction; to impose order upon; orderly or prescribed conduct or pattern of behavior. That doesn't sound too hard does it? I want to train you in new habits that maximize your effort and health. It takes order and a pattern of behavior. I'll give you the prescription, and with the right motivation, I know you'll happily follow it with the promise of healthily attained permanent weight loss. Well, the last set of ab crunches may make you forget the "happily" part, but it will be worth it!

I have established that everyone is different metabolically, and therefore, this chart may not be a perfect fit for a few readers. The goal is to lose one to two pounds of body fat per week and this chart was created for the general population with a moderate activity level. You may lose five to seven pounds the

(Figure 2:3) The Diet Doc Rx (Personal Macronutrient Range)

Height	Men: (Grams per day)	Women:
Under 5'		
Protein	100 - 120	60 - 80
Carbohydrates	120 - 150	80 - 110
Fat	35 - 40	20 - 25
(Calories)	(1,195 - 1,440)	(740 - 985)
5' - 5'4"		
Protein	110 - 130	70 - 90
Carbohydrates	130 - 160	90 - 120
Fat	40 - 45	25 - 30
(Calories)	(1,320 - 1,565)	(865 - 1,110)
5'5" - 5'8"		
Protein	120 - 140	80 - 100
Carbohydrates	140 - 170	100 - 130
Fat	45 - 50	30 - 35
(Calories)	(1,445 - 1,690)	(990 - 1,235)
5'9" - 6'		
Protein	130 - 150	90 - 110
Carbohydrates	150 - 180	110 - 140
Fat	50 - 55	35 - 40
(Calories)	(1,570 - 1,815)	(1,115 - 1,360)
6'1" - 6'4"		
Protein	140 - 160	100 - 120
Carbohydrates	160 - 190	120 - 150
Fat	55 - 60	40 - 45
(Calories)	(1,695 - 1,940)	(1,240 - 1,485)

first week due to water loss, but one to two pounds each week thereafter is the goal. If, despite following your totals perfectly, eating the best food selections as described, and using the methods in this book, you are not obtaining the desired results, you may need to make an adjustment. First, if you are not losing weight fast enough (one to two pounds per week) make sure you're eating at the low end of your macronutrient range. If you are losing too rapidly, make sure you're

eating at the high end. If you're still losing too fast, add 25 grams of

carbohydrates to your daily totals for a week and reassess your results. Keep

adding until you are losing at the desired rate. If you are still losing too slowly

even at the low end of your suggested chart totals, drop your daily intake of carbs

by 10 grams daily for a week and reassess. If necessary, repeat this until you are

losing weight at the appropriate rate.

What to Expect the First Week

As briefly mentioned, your body has many sources of energy to draw

from. As anyone lowers calorie intake below what is necessary (basal metabolic

rate), the caloric deficit must be made up from somewhere. Though we would all

like it to be body fat that is used, there is actually a percentage of energy taken

from almost every available source. The most readily available is blood sugar and

then liver glycogen (stored sugar). These are dynamic, easy-to-access energy

stores that are immediately used when needed.

(Figure 2:4) The First Step

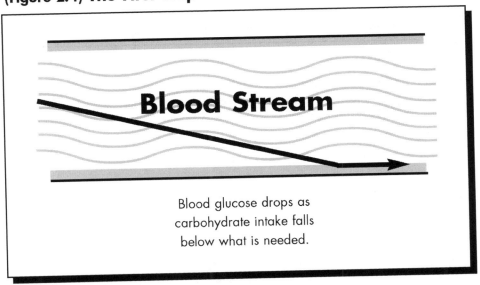

Blood glucose drops as
carbohydrate intake falls
below what is needed.

Muscle glycogen is a large area of stored energy but its primary purpose is

for muscle contraction and work and is therefore not as easily retrieved for

Metabolic Transformation in Action

My life-changing experience with Dr. Joe Klemczewski has been a blessing of untold proportions! I have no doubt whatsoever that he was purposely placed in my life to bring me out of the spiraling downfall of my body's physical health as well as my lagging mental and emotional spirit.

Growing up, throughout my twenties, and even into my mid-thirties, I had always been the envied one who could eat anything and never gain a pound. It was quite a blow to my ego when I started to see the pounds slowly (at first) starting to accumulate. I tried to rationalize that this was normal. After all, I was getting older, right? I went from weighing no more than 120 to around 140 pounds. You need a little extra weight as you get older, others would tell me.

Then, health problems started to flare up – gallbladder removal, female/hormonal problems, back problems, etc. I was getting a bleak picture of the aging process – and the numbers on the scale continued to climb...

The first time I heard of Joe was when my school district hired him to speak to the entire district staff about health and nutrition. Joe has a special ability and talent for taking his vast knowledge of the human body and nutrition and bringing it to a level of understanding that everyone can comprehend. I was extremely impressed and interested, but in my mind I was only slightly overweight at 160 pounds. Others assured me I was fine – but did I feel fine? The numbers on the scale continued to climb...

The next time I heard about Joe was in my doctor's office, Dr. J. Scott Uloth, to whom, by the way, I am eternally grateful. At this point I need to express how Dr. Uloth has been a rock for me during some of the most difficult times of my life. On December 1, 2003, it was necessary for me to have a complete hysterectomy. On December 29 of that same month, my mother passed away unexpectedly, although she had recently been diagnosed with lung cancer. Ten months later, my mother-in-law died suddenly of a massive heart attack. Dr. Uloth listened, talked with me, and helped me through those difficult times. Words can never express my complete gratitude, Dr. Uloth. You are awesome! During this visit, I commented to Dr. Uloth about his own weight loss and overall look of good health. He began to talk to me enthusiastically about Dr. Joe and the help and encouragement he had been provided on his journey back to a healthy lifestyle. He gave me Joe's number and we continued my appointment for back and joint pain. At 174 pounds, the numbers on the scale continued to climb...

continued ⟶

Metabolic Transformation in Action

March, 2004...Once again, I am at Dr. Uloth's office and I am once again running the gamut of aches, pains, illness, and emotions. I compliment Dr. Uloth on looking exceedingly healthy and trim. He, as usual, listened to me patiently, asked questions and looked over my chart. We dealt with my current complaint, of course, and then he broached the subject of my weight gain. My weight at that time was up to, I believe, 204 pounds. I had gained about 40 pounds from mid-December 2003 to March of 2004. We talked about the causes of the weight gain, both physical and emotional. At the age of 42, soon to be 43 years old, I had never felt so out of control in my life. I was trapped in an unhealthy body that didn't seem to respond to any of my many attempts to lose weight and improve my health. Dr. Uloth again mentioned all the positive effects of his work with Dr. Joe. I told him I was most definitely interested, but that it was an extremely busy time for me both at work and at home. I would be getting in touch with Dr. Joe after school was out in May. I left feeling more hopeful than I had in a while, but the numbers on the scale continued to climb...

On Wednesday, May 25, 2005, I had my first personal meeting with Dr. Joe. My weight had climbed to an unbelievable all-time high of 215 pounds! I was in an embarrassed, emotional state of mind and Dr. Joe had a very calming, reassuring manner. He talked with me for about two hours, explaining the importance of nutrition in weight loss, learning about my eating and exercise habits, my lifestyle, etc. I was so excited because I understood what he was saying! I'm a schoolteacher, so I don't consider myself ignorant, but he made health, nutrition, and complex physiology fit together and make sense in a way I had never understood before. I left his office with a sense of purpose, determination, and hope for my future well-being. My journey had begun – and on that day, the numbers on the scale quit climbing.

Nutrition has been the most important factor in my weight loss. I keep a daily food journal that allows me to see in just a glance if my food intake of protein, carbs, and fat is appropriate. I also have managed to work regular exercise into my lifestyle – a feat I had previously claimed was impossible due to lack of valuable time. Joe is always available to me via e-mail for questions, concerns, and most importantly, encouragement. I immediately noticed a huge upsurge in my energy level and that I wasn't experiencing the hunger and mood swings that I had regularly experienced before. I knew in my heart that this time I would succeed!

continued ⟶

Metabolic Transformation in Action

It wasn't long until friends and family began asking me questions: "You've lost weight! What are you doing?" and "You seem different? What's going on?" It wasn't just the weight they were noticing. It was the difference in my demeanor, attitude, and general outlook on life. My husband and children could see that I was finally returning to the way I used to be – the wife and mom they had been missing so much.

I have tried many, many other weight-loss facilities and programs. They offered counseling sessions, encouraged food journaling, and some even told me exactly what to eat. I managed to lose weight for a while, but something was missing. I always went back to my old habits and gained it back, plus some. After working with Joe, I believe the missing "something" is the fact that he truly cares and believes in you so much, you simply cannot fail! He goes the extra miles it takes to make sure you understand and can succeed. You learn to believe in your own abilities and that translates in to all aspects of your life. When I said life-changing experience at the beginning, I meant life-changing, not just the weight.

As of November 30, 2005 I have lost 54 pounds! I still have a lot of weight to lose, but I have no doubt in my mind that I will lose the weight and keep it off for life. With Dr. Joe's help, I have completely changed my way of thinking about food. In October, my family and I went to Florida for a 10-day vacation and I did not gain an ounce. Believe me, that was a first!

My spiraling journey continues onward and upward now, but the numbers on the scales are going down! Thank you, Dr. Joe! Thank you, Dr. Uloth! I am a different person – the person I need to be for myself and for my family – because you both took the time and effort to care.

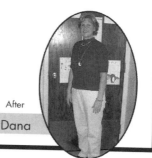

After

Dana

maintenance calorie needs. Between meals, body fat is released from body fat cells, but only as much as is needed. So, if you follow the path, this paragraph will be monumental to your understanding. Your food intake is now precise and consistent so that you will get precise and consistent results. The total amount of calories is moderately lower than your body needs on a daily basis so that it requires a secondary source of calories. The first place your body is going to access is blood sugar, liver glycogen, and a moderate amount of available muscle glycogen (especially if you work out). The Diet Doc Rx chart is

(Figure 2:5) Step Two

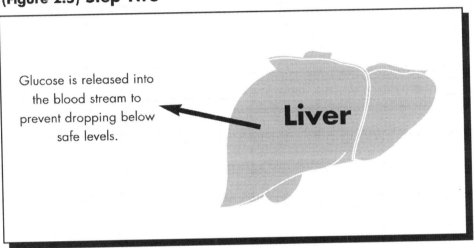

Glucose is released into the blood stream to prevent dropping below safe levels.

Liver

designed to take a large portion of the caloric deficit from carbohydrates so that as you continue using blood sugar and glycogen, you will eventually (within two to four days) be as depleted as your brain will safely allow. This is a large portion of the deficit we're creating, but it in no way makes it a low-carbohydrate diet. Blood sugar levels are critical to the brain and body so your brain won't let you go too far without throwing a tantrum. At this point, you'll feel hungry, possibly weak and shaky, maybe tired, and some will even get a headache. Since this is not a low-carb diet, this phase will be brief and is a rite of passage that leads to success. You now have reached a level of carbohydrate depletion that opens a door to significant body-fat loss. If you give in to the hunger at this point, you'll refill your muscle and liver glycogen as well as your blood stream glucose (sugar) and you'll have to <u>start</u> <u>over</u>. Unfortunately, this is a pattern of many dieters. Three or four days go well, and then a binge sends them back to the starting block both physically and mentally. What happens in reality is that they deplete and replete carb stores without much alteration in body fat and though they really are eating well 80% of the time, they don't lose weight.

If, however, you stay within your macronutrient range through this tough day of being moderately carb depleted, a great accomplishment takes place.

(Figure 2:6) Final Step in Carb Depletion

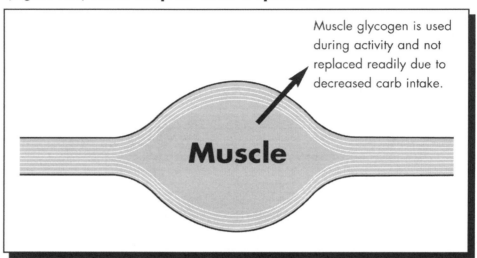

Since you're not giving in to the carb cravings, your brain is forced into plan B. Plan B is that since you're not providing more glucose from your diet, your body has to find another source. I can't emphasize enough how amazing the design of our body is. Two things will now happen that allows for immediate and consistent body fat loss. Body fat cells start releasing fatty acids and glycerol, the products of stored body fat. Once in the blood stream, some is used directly by certain types of cells for energy (lipolysis) while more actually gets converted into glucose. This mechanism is called gluconeogenesis, literally the creation of new glucose. Now blood sugar levels come back up to a consistent level so energy returns and hunger decreases. As a matter of fact there is almost a euphoric rise in energy and a marked decrease in lethargy throughout the day due to the consistency in blood sugar. This is real energy; not the temporary caffeine or sugar high that leaves you jittery, dazed, and then asleep! As long as you're consistent with your suggested food intake totals, you're now making up the majority of the caloric deficit through the mechanism of turning your body fat into new carbohydrates. It isn't difficult to understand the purpose of this design is so that we can survive for long periods of time by accessing these stored calories in the form of body fat if necessary. By learning how to effectively take advantage of this inherent survival mechanism you're going to lose body fat permanently without the suffering fad diets often cause.

(Figure 2:7) The Breaking Point

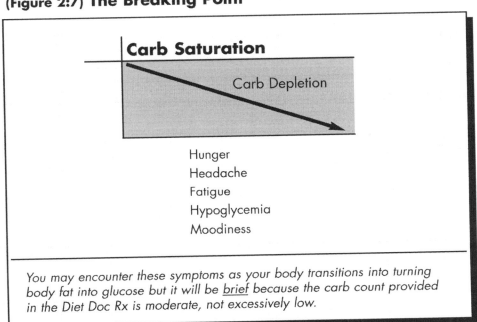

Carb Saturation

Carb Depletion

Hunger
Headache
Fatigue
Hypoglycemia
Moodiness

You may encounter these symptoms as your body transitions into turning body fat into glucose but it will be <u>*brief*</u> *because the carb count provided in the Diet Doc Rx is moderate, not excessively low.*

Another way of explaining it is that the brain needs a constant supply of glucose in the blood stream. To make sure glucose levels aren't too high or too low, the brain directs the pancreas to produce more glucagon (to raise blood sugar) or insulin (to store blood sugar). Fat loss or fat gain <u>isn't</u> the primary goal of the body with food; it's an indirect effect based on what hormone – glucagon or insulin – is present most often. Too much carbohydrate in one meal results in insulin being dominant and we're in a storage mode. Too little carbohydrate and we're in a retrieving mode. So why not eliminate carbs completely? More on that critical question coming up. When too much carbohydrate is present and insulin runs rampant, we store the glucose in our liver and muscle, (meaning we have to once again deplete that carbohydrate to begin burning body fat maximally), and some of the blood glucose gets directly pulled into fat cells and stored as fat. Note the study regarding yo-yo dieting.

One thing to keep in mind is that each gram of glycogen holds approximately three times its weight in water. A by-product of cellular metabolism is also water. So, the first week of decreasing your body's level of stored carbohydrates and beginning the process of losing body fat will result in a large amount of water loss. It isn't uncommon for someone to lose five to eight pounds in the first week. The second week's weight loss will be a truer reflection of how much body fat is being lost.

Can't I Have Just One Piece of Pizza?

Here's the best news of the book so far. You get a "splurge" meal. Not a splurge day and not a lay-on-the-couch-moaning splurge meal after visiting every buffet in town. If you're on track with your personal Diet Doc Rx and you're losing at the pace described, you can and should have one meal per week where you enjoy foods you've been avoiding as "not the best weight-loss foods." Have a couple pieces of pizza and a dessert. Have a steak and potato and even a dinner roll. Eat a moderate amount and enjoy it without guilt. You'll be replacing your normal dinner and possibly a snack, so the calorie overage isn't that much; perhaps just barely over your metabolic rate. This does several things. First, you need that boost in food intake so your body doesn't continue in a chronic calorie deficit for too long. Recall the studies showing how fast and how far your metabolism can fall. Secondly, you get a nice break from the deficit and the feeling of being deprived. You may not think you need these breaks. You're tough, right? But chronic depletion can sneak up on you and having this pause only makes you less prone to binging, and as I said, you really do need it physiologically for long-term progress. Some nice side effects are that you get used to eating "normal" or "bad" food, however you want to describe it, without going overboard in volume and you have the flexibility of a floating "meal off" to use for special occasions. Plan your splurge meal for that birthday party or that football game. I would always keep this in play and if it slows your progress down, cut your daily amount of carbs just a little to be able to keep moving forward with the splurge meal.

CHAPTER TWO KEY POINTS

• • • • ▶ 1) Correct nutrition can raise your metabolism to help achieve weight loss.

• • • • ▶ 2) The right amount of food per day is the first and most important step in achieving permanent and predictable weight loss through raising your metabolism.

• • • • ▶ 3) You must follow your macronutrient totals consistently to achieve this predictable body fat loss – take your Rx!

• • • • ▶ 4) It may be necessary to adjust your macronutrient totals.

• • • • ▶ 5) After two to four days, be prepared to feel hungry, tired, and possibly get a headache as your body prepares to begin converting body fat into glucose. Stay on course; it will only last one day at the most.

• • • • ▶ 6) Be patient with the amount of information you are learning. It will continue to make more sense as you keep reading.

Chapter Three

MEAL STRUCTURING

Meal Portions

Now that you have established how much food you need per day, how are you to structure this food into your daily meals and snacks? This question is far more important than you might think. You can actually gain or lose weight eating the exact same amount of food just by changing how you schedule your meals during the day.

There is a limit to how much food your body can effectively digest, metabolize, and absorb at one time. If you eat too much at a meal, some of that food ends up stored as new body fat. So even if you're eating the right amount of food per day, you could be working against yourself by storing new body fat at certain meals. At best, this could slow your progress; at worst, it could negate any progress at all. This pattern can result from our culture's typical way of eating: skip breakfast, grab a candy bar or burger at lunch, and then start supper in the kitchen and extend it until bedtime. Recall from chapter two that in creating a calorie deficit we first draw dominantly from intermediate energy, mostly stored glycogen from the liver and muscle. Only when we use most of what is stored there do we switch over in a larger way to stored body fat. If we constantly eat larger meals, even though we stay calorically in line for the day, we have periods of time where we cause insulin to be released in too high of amounts, restore glycogen, and we move out of the accelerated body fat burning mode. Not only does this style of eating promote consuming too much at one time, it also means going for long periods of time without eating. This brings up another problem.

Once digestion, absorption, and metabolism of consumed nutrients have slowed and stopped after a meal, your body starts using stored energy. If you go too long without eating, your metabolic processes taper to conserve energy. So, if you eat only a couple of large meals per day, your body starts converting the excess food from large meals into body fat at the same time that glycogen is being restored. During the long periods between meals, your metabolism slows down. Essentially, you have created a downward spiral of storing new body fat and then made it more difficult to lose due to a slowing metabolism. Furthermore, you will be prone to storing more body fat at the next meal due to the hormonal changes. Talk about a vicious cycle! The act of digesting food and the subsequent increase of cellular metabolism that takes place is actually the greatest way to affect long-term calorie burning. The more times you eat, the higher your metabolism rises within your genetic limit. So, be sure to not skip your snacks.

Skipping a meal or snack once in awhile isn't going to send your metabolism tumbling. Making it a way of life will. The biggest reason that smaller meals work better is so that you don't store extra body fat like you would at larger meals and your metabolism is actually increased every time you eat. If you can raise your metabolism more frequently with smaller meals and you're not storing new fat at those meals, you're in fat-loss overdrive!

Power Spacing

Five to even eight small meals and snacks per day should be a goal. By frequently eating meals small enough so they are completely used and not stored as body fat, you can keep your metabolism charged to maximal levels. Sometimes you may not be hungry for that scheduled snack, but keep your eye on your schedule. If you skip one and then can't eat for another couple of hours, hunger may drive you to binge or eat what you didn't have planned.

Several factors can make it easy to design your meal spacing plan. First and foremost, divide the quantity of macronutrients logically, not necessarily perfectly. Two to three meals per day should be solid, normal meals much the same as you may currently eat, except in the right amounts. (Food choices and actual meals with macronutrient ratios will be discussed in later chapters.) The remaining two to three meals per day will be smaller snacks. Try to eat your meals or snacks every three to four hours. I can hear many of you grumbling, "I don't have time to eat that many times a day!" Be honest, though; we can all sip

AVERAGE JOE PHYSIOLOGY

The Dynamic Duo – Hormones that is

Believe it or not, gaining or losing body fat is merely a symptom of a delicate balance of hormones in your body. As you now know, insulin causes glucose (carbohydrates) to be stored and glucagon instigates fat loss. Insulin stores; glucagon retrieves. Insulin creates fat stores; glucagon removes stored body fat. In a normal state of balance in the body, three times more insulin is present in the blood stream compared to glucagon. The fact that there is 50 million times greater amounts of blood glucose than these hormones combined, shows how powerful they are in small amounts. Subtle swings in either direction cause major metabolic changes. Consider a visual illustration of a teeter-totter: glucagon on one side, insulin the other. When insulin increases above its normal levels, the body starts storing more energy than normal. If glucagon starts increasing, energy will be harvested within the body. Studies show that when carbohydrates are decreased, glucagon concentration increases. Through a cascade of events, body fat is used as energy as an end result. When meal intervals are well-planned, overt increases in carbohydrates, and therefore insulin, are easier to avoid. Over the course of a day, a week, and a month, one would spend more time with higher blood levels of glucagon compared to insulin and would have lost more body fat even with a similar overall calorie intake. This gives you quite an edge in dieting. You're literally working with your body instead of against it.

on a protein shake or stop for five minutes to grab a snack even if we're still working. This is another reason to plan ahead. Meal spacing is second only to The Diet Doc Rx in importance if you want to achieve the safest, most efficient weight loss. This is a difficult, habitual shift for most people, but it is <u>critical</u>.

Having provided an overview of the importance of meal spacing, I want you to know exactly why this step is so important. Recall from chapter two that your body is essentially in a constant state of metabolic storage or retrieval. Blood nutrient levels are being kept steady by the work of virtually every system of your body. After a meal, the body is working to digest and distribute nutrients in a pattern based on priority. Seemingly frantic processes are occurring to keep the body functioning at its highest level. As those critical needs are being met,

(Figure 3:1) **Power Spacing**

6:00 a.m.	Breakfast
9:00 a.m.	Snack
12:00 p.m.	Lunch
3:00 p.m.	Snack
6:00 p.m.	Supper
9:00 p.m.	Small snack (optional)

however, excess food is quickly stored, since it is not needed at that particular time. Remember, the body is built for survival. What it doesn't need now, it will store to use later. Excess fat in a meal can be stored directly as body fat right out of the bloodstream and excess carbohydrates will be converted into triglycerides and also stuffed into fat cells. Both of these processes will be discussed in depth in upcoming chapters.

The bottom line is that too much food in one meal will create new body fat on the premise that your body will be able to use it later. This happens constantly even to people whose weight is very stable. We store a little body fat and then use it between meals. Those of us that carry more weight than is healthy, though, are walking reminders that we're storing more at those meals than we're ultimately using. The answer isn't to wait longer between meals; the answer is to not overeat at meals and stop the storage process before it starts. This is critically important because we store body fat much easier than we use it. Once digestion and absorption are complete after a meal and our blood sugar levels start to lower, we now have to work our way through the newly stored glycogen in the liver and the blood lipids (fat) before we start using a larger portion of stored body fat. If we overeat we may never even get to that level of working our way through our stores before we eat again and restart the process.

Conversely, if we eat meals that contain correct amounts of protein, carbohydrates, and fat to allow our body to function optimally, we increase the likelihood of not storing anything new as fat, and instead spend more time between meals in a retrieval mode of burning stored body fat for energy. You'll find that you're ready for that next meal even if you're not used to eating frequently. You can quickly create a pattern of stability in your metabolism that keeps blood nutrient levels from fluctuating wildly, energy levels high, and body fat usage constant. The alternative of eating larger, less frequent meals will lead to slower weight loss, potential weight gain, and fatigue.

Keep in mind that there really isn't a perfect ratio. I often get asked if meals should be exactly the same size and spaced exactly at certain intervals. If you're that obsessive compulsive, life itself has probably given you an anxiety disorder and I don't want to add to it! It actually is easy to assume that there must be a perfect formula since nutrition is a science, but your daily activity, schedule, and energy expenditure create a ton of metabolic diversity. Depending on your daily living activities and exercise, you may have different metabolic needs and hunger patterns on different days. It's important that you allow yourself the flexibility for your meals to vary in size, time, and content day to day without thinking you're failing. You'll gradually find some habits become mainstays and other meals you may change often. The greatest thing about not being locked into someone else's food plan is that the freedom leads to thinking on your feet. You learn to succeed by using your brain. A novel idea in this era of cookie-cutter diet books!

The Convenience Factor

Eating five to eight times a day poses a scheduling challenge to most people. However, once you have adopted this new way of eating, you will have so much more energy that you'll never want to revert to your past meal pattern. Gone will be the temporary, artificial energy brought on by sugar and caffeine, and it will be replaced by constant energy from steady blood glucose levels. Eating small, frequent meals keeps nutrients flowing into your body, which is the cornerstone of good health and weight management. Blood sugar, nitrogen (protein), and blood lipid (fat) levels all stay more uniform via small meals.

Metabolic Transformation in Action

A few months after I turned 53, I got really tired of the fact that too many of my clothes were fitting tightly, even though I had been jogging, riding my bike, and "watching" what I ate. The weight on my 5'6" frame just seemed to stay around 165 no matter what I did. This was 20 pounds more than I weighed just 10 years earlier. (I had lost 5 pounds on a popular plan when I was 50, but like almost everyone else I know who tried it, I had gained it all back.)

One day I happened to catch Dr. Joe on a local TV show. Having recognized him from church, I called him and set up an hour consultation. Joe's approach to nutrition and good body stewardship has since affected my life very dramatically. In fact, the change has been so dynamic in me, it is a physical equivalent to the spiritual rebirth the Bible speaks of.

Dr. Joe simply gave me an eating plan to make my body start burning stored fat. Within 25 days, I lost 10 pounds of it, and in less than 5 months I was down to 135. My weight has remained between 131 and 135 for 2 years – along with the 30" waist I had in high school!!! My energy and stamina multiplied. I just feel like a new and different person. Medically speaking, my trigycerides have dropped from 249 to 88, my HDL ("good" cholesterol) rose from 46 to 68, and my LDL ("bad" cholesterol) dropped from 122 to 98.

On the Metabolic Transformation plan...
• I did not get the "munchies." I just got hungry for a meal of real food.
• I didn't feel like I was sacrificing anything, food-wise.
• I didn't eat any "weird" food like rice cakes or celery bread or grapefruit rind.
• I was not hungry for the cookies, cake, pie, etc. that had been one of my "basic food groups" all my life. It did not bother me to pass by the many sweets that I frequently encounter during the course of a day.
• I don't have any plan or desire to go back to my old eating habits. I love/enjoy what I am eating now, and could eat this way for the rest of my life.

Part of Joe's strategy is strengthening the body through weight training. This has been extremely invigorating. With the newfound energy that intelligent eating gives me, I am able to do a vigorous work out 3 times a week, and so at 55 am in the best shape of my life! Last year I set personal

continued ——→

Metabolic Transformation in Action

lifetime speed records for running the 5K, and was also able to climb 5,235 feet to the ridge crest of Mt. Whitney (13,600 ft) and back in one day.

I have come to realize that an hour of vigorous exercise is NOT a waste of time "when you should be doing something more important." It is tuning up your body so you can accomplish in a more efficient way what God needs you to. The hour I spend lifting weights or running I get back in the one less hour of sleep I need, a more alert mind, and relaxed body.

I know that there are many weight-loss theories and programs; however, I can't help thinking there is something very unique and permanent about Metabolic Transformation. And you won't find anyone with a keener mind who is more concerned about your total well being than Dr. Joe. The surge in my self-confidence that he gave me has resulted in positive effects too numerous to mention. Thanks a million, Joe!

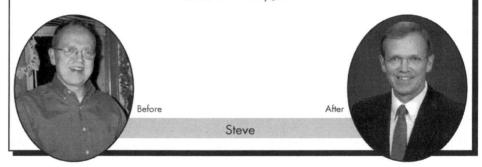

Before · Steve · After

Everyone has experienced lulls (and even crashes) in energy during the day. With well-spaced meals, these lulls will disappear and be replaced with steady, high energy levels.

You can easily overcome meal scheduling challenges with good planning. Meal replacement drinks ("protein shakes") and high-quality food ("energy") bars can be very good, convenient snack choices. Low-glycemic fruit, yogurt, and many other whole-food choices are also easy to fit into your daily routine. If there is such a thing as meal timing and quantity perfection, you would still have a problem sustaining that "perfect" schedule every day. The good news is that you don't have to. Some days are understandably going to be wild, on the run, and impossible to do as well as you want. The first thing to always consider is your ultimate goal. If you're in a hurry, don't use it as an excuse to stop for a cookie dough milk shake because you "didn't have time for anything else." It's always better to grab a healthy carb source, like a piece of fruit, even if it causes you to be out of your macronutrient range for the day (because you likely may be low on protein or fat). So the extra carbs won't do that much damage. It may not be a "perfect" day, but it's not a diet catastrophe.

Stay well-armed with good food and plan ahead to make sure you can eat when you should eat, but when all else fails, get the best alternative you can and regroup. This is where your log book comes in handy. If you have a running total of what you've consumed for the day, I guarantee you'll make better choices on the spot. Even with no one looking over your shoulder, it will be rewarding for you to know that you're staying on your plan even in a pinch. These small daily successes will make you a confident weight-loss warrior.

CHAPTER THREE KEY POINTS

1) *Too much food at one meal leads to new body fat storage.*

2) *Too much time between meals slows the metabolism.*

3) *Five to seven small meals/snacks can maximize metabolic rate and keep body fat loss consistent.*

4) *Well-planned and spaced meals will lead to steady, high energy levels throughout the entire day.*

5) *Convenience is very important. Plan ahead to make sure you can eat when you should.*

6) *An ounce of preparation is worth a pound on your waistline.*

Chapter Four

CARBOHYDRATES

Friend or Foe?

Chapters two and three answered structural questions: how much should I eat, and how should I create and space my meals? Now the discussion moves directly to food. As discussed previously, food is divided into three main macronutrients: protein, carbohydrates, and fat. Each is dramatically different both in structure and function. A calorie isn't just a calorie. A calorie is a unit of energy, a measurement. One gram of carbohydrate equals four calories as does one gram of protein. Fat, often called a more "dense" nutrient, has nine calories per gram. Even though each calorie is the same unit of energy, the effect on your body's chemistry and function is quite different depending on its source (protein, carbs, or fat). That is why some methods of weight loss are more effective than others. Each macronutrient will be covered in its own chapter. I'll begin with the most controversial.

Many dietitians and nutritionists have elevated carbohydrates to an almost untouchable level of nutritional deity. For decades, dieticians devised weight-loss schemes with carbohydrates at the center of the diets. Until recently, commercials bragged about how cereals are full of "nutritious carbohydrates." Witness now everyone's change in language to "whole grains" since the low-carb craze has made "carbohydrate" a dirty word.

Long before nutrition was a studied science, it was understood that athletes needed more fuel – more calories – to support their training. Like now, carbohydrates were the most abundant, least expensive, most convenient, and usually best-tasting food. Since athletes were observed consuming many more carbohydrates than anyone else and had physiques that were admired by all, the conclusion was drawn that eating carbs was the way to go. My more science-oriented readers (like my organic chemistry professor who stained my transcript with the only "C" that appears in over 10 years of college meandering – I still haven't forgiven him), may already be able to conclude that correlation does not equal causation. Athletes may be able to eat a great deal of carbohydrates and not gain body fat due to their intense levels of training, but what about those of us who don't train as hard? And just because athletes may "get away" with eating too many carbs because of their energy expenditure, does that mean it's the best nutrition even for them?

AVERAGE JOE PHYSIOLOGY

Double Your Fat Loss

In a review of isocaloric diet studies (diets that compare the same amount of calories but with different ratios of protein, carbohydrates, and fat) it is difficult to find outcomes different than was found by the International Journal of Obesity. Studies were reviewed and compared that controlled subject group calories at 1,000 and were divided into higher-carbohydrate/low-fat groups and higher-fat/low-carbohydrate groups. Other studies were reviewed using the same type of nutrient ratios but even higher calories. The groups on lower carbohydrates, but the same amount of overall calories, lost 43% more weight. That is a strong indictment against high-carb diets, but not necessarily an endorsement of no-carb diets. As you will see, carbs have their place and taking their elimination to an extreme will cause extreme problems. Carbohydrates are a key variable, but knowing what the correct level to decrease them to depends on several factors.

Of course, the inevitable response to one extreme is always the opposite extreme, so it didn't take long for no-carbohydrate diets to creep onto the scene like a brain fog. To answer these questions and cut our way through a still raging controversy, let's turn to metabolic physiology. (Or, if I've lost you already, take a break and turn to the sports page or the comics for awhile and then come back. I'll wait.) Once you understand exactly what happens inside your body when you eat different foods, you will be able to discern good nutrition from bad.

(Figure 4:1) Carbohydrate Digestion

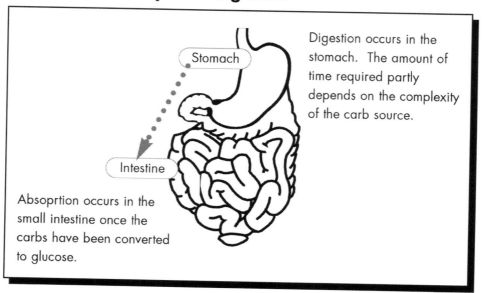

Stomach

Digestion occurs in the stomach. The amount of time required partly depends on the complexity of the carb source.

Intestine

Absoprtion occurs in the small intestine once the carbs have been converted to glucose.

Carbohydrate Structure and Function

Carbohydrates provide most of the energy for our bodies most of the time. Because they require the least amount of energy to break down, carbohydrates are the easiest of the macronutrients to digest and be converted to glucose. Carb sources are loosely described as sugars, starches, or fibers, and these are commonly described as simple and complex carbohydrates. We typically think of simple carbohydrates as junk food, like soda and candy, and complex carbs as whole foods, like potatoes, pasta, and bread. This type of categorization leads to the false assumption that a particular food is either good or bad when actually there is more of a continuum that allows detailed comparison. Good, better, best, bad, and/or worse may be more appropriate ways of describing carb choices once you understand how they compare to one another and how they affect your body. (Didn't Jerry Springer do a show on this: bad carbs and the women who love them?)

Glucose is the smallest sugar molecule possible. It is the form of sugar that the human body uses for energy. Whatever form of carbohydrate you consume, the end result of digestion is glucose. There are, however, many forms of carbohydrates, and the pathway of digestion that leads to glucose is what can affect our energy levels, mental acuity, physical functioning, and even athletic performance.

You may recognize the names of various forms of sugar: glucose, lactose, fructose, maltose, dextrose, sucrose, and so on. Each one of these carbohydrates has a different level of molecular complexity. Those that are made primarily of glucose are easy and quick to digest since most of the carbs are already in the smallest possible form. (For dieters, that's bad.) Those with a more complex molecular structure are harder to digest and take longer to move through the digestion process. (That's good!) The *Glycemic Index* (Fig. 4:8) is a scale that ranks carbohydrate foods by comparing their structures. It reveals the simplicity or complexity of the sugar, starch, and fiber that make up the macronutrient called carbohydrates.

(Figure 4:2) Insulin Reaction

When too many carbs, or carbs which are too simple (high-glycemic), are consumed, blood sugar rises rapidly.

Insulin released

(Normal blood sugar range)

Just to Make Sure You're Still Awake

Two caveats that need explanation are fiber and sugar alcohols. The popularity of low-carb diets have led people to believe that fiber and sugar alcohol is "free" and doesn't need counted. Fiber, though it is digested slower, is a carbohydrate. Any that doesn't get digested in the stomach can be actually broken down in the large intestine. So, while fibrous carbs are good, healthy sources, they are still, and must be counted as, carbohydrates.

An interesting carbohydrate source that the FDA hasn't classified firmly (gee, the government confusing us? Who'd of thought?) is sugar alcohol, or polyphenols. Used in some baked products, and very prevalent in protein/energy bars, sugar alcohol (usually in the form of glycerine or glycerol) is actually part of a fat molecule. Being calorically similar to a carbohydrate, but structurally coming from a fat molecule, and the fact that it is digested very slowly without a fast rise in blood sugar (did I mention this was confusing?) originally led the FDA to not even require listing it on the label. Talk about denial – we don't know what it is, so we'll just ignore it? Whether due to lobbying efforts by the low-carb food producers or due to the reduced danger to diabetics (since it doesn't cause a fast rise in blood sugar) sugar alcohol was allowed to fly under the radar. When the outcry was loud enough, the FDA started requiring them to be rightly listed in "total carbohydrates" on the label, but they continue to allow fiber and polyphenols to be deducted to create a new category: net carbs. Again, these carbs are there and need to be counted. Don't deduct fiber and ignore "net carb" counts; track "total carbohydrates."

Alcoholic beverages are similar but don't even (as of yet) provide the courtesy of the "net carb" label. Look at any low-carb, light beer and you'll find near-zero protein and fat counts, a low carbohydrate count, but calories listed at a much higher level than if you did the math. (Protein and carbs have four calories per gram and fat has nine.) The "missing calories" are carbs not counted – sugar alcohol. Wine and hard liquor are roughly four grams of carbs per ounce, though they'll be often listed as just one. Those light beers that you think you've been downing at a cost of only 7 to 10 grams of carbs are really about 20 to 25. I know I didn't make any friends with that one!

Back to Business

When you consume a high-glycemic index carbohydrate such as white bread, a banana, a baked potato, soda, candy, etc., you are consuming a carbohydrate that is primarily glucose. Little digestion needs to take place with these foods. They pass through the stomach quickly and enter the small intestine. Absorption occurs in the small intestine, and since so much glucose enters so fast, uptake is rapid. Your brain closely monitors your blood sugar levels, and such a rapid increase triggers your pancreas to release the hormone insulin. Remember, insulin is the storage hormone that shuttles blood glucose where it is needed.

Most of us aren't glycogen-depleted (short of stored glucose), so our muscles and livers usually contain plenty of glucose for fuel. Depending on how many carbohydrates you consume at one time, chances are you will have too much blood sugar and nowhere to store it. Your already high level of circulating insulin causes your liver to convert the blood sugar into triglycerides (fat) to be ultimately stored. Insulin also triggers body fat cells to simply pull excess glucose in to be converted directly into body fat.

(Figure 4:3) Carbohydrate Conversion to Body Fat

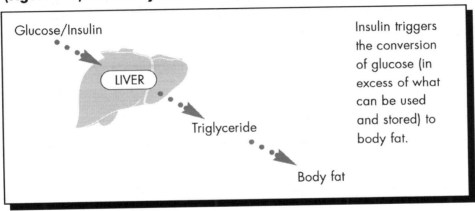

Glucose/Insulin

LIVER

Triglyceride

Body fat

Insulin triggers the conversion of glucose (in excess of what can be used and stored) to body fat.

None of the aforementioned high-glycemic carb sources have fat in them, but a large portion of the carbs can be converted to body fat due to the effect of insulin. Unfortunately, the problems don't stop there. Be it by storage, utilization, or by fat conversion, your blood glucose levels return to normal and your brain tells your pancreas to stop releasing insulin. However, even with the process stopped, a certain amount of insulin remains active in the bloodstream until it is "used up." This means more blood sugar will be removed, dropping it below the normal level. A blood sugar level that's too low will leave you tired as in the case of the after-lunch dosing behind the desk. Even worse, your brain sends out powerful hormonal messengers to signal hunger. I'm sure you've experienced eating something and being even hungrier a short while later. Too much of a drop and you can have more severe symptoms such as hypoglyecemia. Have you ever ended up weak, shaky, and starving just 30 or 60 minutes after eating?

(Figure 4:4) Insulin Overcompensation

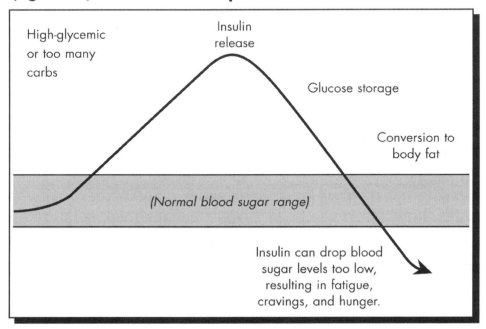

The tragedy of this whole process is it takes you from bad to worse in body composition, energy levels, and health in one fell swoop. You either block body fat loss or store new body fat with a "fat-free" food. You then end up tired and so hungry with carbohydrate cravings that you eat a similar meal and start the process all over again. This is an extremely powerful biochemical reaction. Massive, seemingly uncontrollable binges are birthed by insulin-induced low blood sugar. Many of us live on this roller coaster and don't realize that we're the ones causing it! "I just have a slow metabolism," or "You just naturally gain more body fat as you get older…" – I know you've used these excuses, and I know you've believed them. It's time to gain control over your nutrition for good.

Falling Off the Wagon

Binging isn't an eating disorder, though it can lead to one. Binging is often rooted in the physiology of dieting too hard. When you sustain too low of a carbohydrate level for too long, your body is going to crave carbs and most of us aren't going to be able to stop eating once we start. It's common but it's devastating. Listen in to an e-mail from a client:

"So...I knew it would not take long before you discovered the real me. I haven't sent you this week's food diary but suffice it to say that it is not good at all. This is me. Unable to stick to clean eating for more than days at a time, disgusted with myself, and firmly believing that it is my destiny to be chubby and miserable all the time. Yet I make these choices. I understand that each time I eat ice cream or chocolate or whatever, that I am making the choice to do so. What I don't know is why I can't seem to correct my behavior. And I don't consider myself one of those people who cheats just to try to get away with as much as possible. No, I try, oh, Lord, how I do try...then I crack and I eat something I shouldn't because I just HAVE TO... then I can't stop so I eat more. Then I feel guilty and disgusted with myself. Then I get into a cycle o,f 'Well, you've already screwed up so if you do it again it doesn't matter.' And I do, which perpetuates the cycle. Then I get really mad at myself and say, 'Okay, get over it, move on, you'll be okay.' And I go great guns and do really well until yet again, after days of pacing around my kitchen looking at food or gazing at the giant cookies at the supermarket, I give in and the self-destruction begins again. 'Well, I screwed up and ate the cookies so if I eat this cake too it doesn't matter.' It doesn't seem to matter how much variation I get, how many carbs or how little, there is stuff I WANT and I can never seem to shake it. And it's very bad when I am at work with all the treats people bring in. I know my choices only hurt my chances of achieving my goal, yet I do it any way. Through weeks and weeks of dieting I tell myself how much I am sacrificing and suffering and I think, 'Why go through all of this and then mess it up for a piece of pie?' But somehow I manage (in the moment) to justify that it won't matter. Am I insane? Am I just a loser?"

Have you been there? I have. There are three critical points I want you to see illustrated in that e-mail. The first is the cycle I mentioned above: if you don't give yourself a chance to move away from the dominance of over-consuming carbohydrates, and if you never get past that "sticking point" and make it into a couple of days of stability, you may stay in that miserable cycle. The second point is that it does take a few days for your body to stabilize and it <u>does</u> get easier. Hunger decreases, cravings decrease, and it's a very noticeable shift. Both of these points are physical. It is sugar withdrawal, and you have to get through it. These biological impulses are going to happen regardless of how

(Figure 4:5) Stable Blood Sugar Through Carbohydrate Management

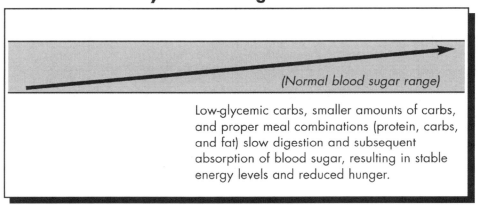

(Normal blood sugar range)

Low-glycemic carbs, smaller amounts of carbs, and proper meal combinations (protein, carbs, and fat) slow digestion and subsequent absorption of blood sugar, resulting in stable energy levels and reduced hunger.

strong- or weak-willed you may be in the moment of temptation. Good meal spacing will help you get through this detox – use it. The last point, though, is your will. During those tough points, it helps to have a sense of righteous indignation – "I'm not putting THAT in my body!" Or a sense of mission and pride – "Being lean means more to me than that cookie! I can do it!!" Avoid having those foods around, ask those around you to help, do anything you think will help, but get beyond this roller coaster and make it easier for yourself. Once you move into a deeper level of body fat metabolism through controlled and consistent carbohydrate intake, stability will be just around the corner.

Stability Can Be Controlled; by You!

Now that you actually <u>understand</u> the physiological problems created by getting outside your ranges (getting too high and spiking your insulin thereby causing fat storage, or getting too low and setting off a hypoglycemic eating binge) you can move to <u>permanent</u> control. You are not a "loser" and you are not "insane," but don't do the "whatever" eating and quit doing "I've already screwed up so I might as well keep going." Those behaviors only lead to greater fat storage. If you must have a treat, don't view yourself as a failure. Everyone loves a treat. I know I sure as heck do! Simply try to make better choices for that treat. Eat in control, keep close to your ranges, and you'll be fine. You are well on your way to understanding and working smarter not harder. Quit putting yourself in a shame spiral and beating yourself up. You <u>can</u> do this. I will further caution you to not let sugary treats become a habit and replace a large portion of your carbohydrate ranges. You might be able to fit 46 grams of carbs from a soda into your daily ranges, but you will be crowding out healthy carb sources such as fruits, vegetables, and whole grains in addition to harming your pancreas and making your body work harder to lose weight. Don't do it. Concentrate on health and the things that will make it easier to succeed.

(Figure 4:6) The Energy Continuum

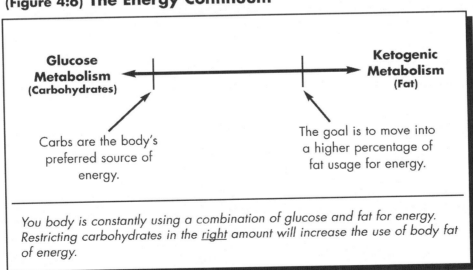

What if you chose a carbohydrate on the other end of the glycemic index, such as a grapefruit, an apple, a bowl of oatmeal, or even a salad? These carb sources have different molecular configurations of glucose. Fructose, cellulose, galactose, etc., are much more complex forms of carbohydrate. When these hit your stomach, digestion takes longer to break them into usable glucose molecules. Since this process takes more time, the molecules enter the small intestine and are absorbed more gradually. Blood sugar levels now rise more slowly, avoiding a major insulin increase. Just by changing the carb source you have decreased the potential for the creation of new body fat, and your energy level rises over the next couple of hours instead of plummeting quickly. Possibly best of all for someone who is dieting, hunger is dramatically reduced because blood glucose levels are stable instead of too low, such as at the end of an insulin rampage.

Think back to our chapter two discussion of the opposite effects of insulin and glucagon. During a new client consultation just last week, my new "student" said, "So keeping insulin low is the whole key?" Though there are so many swirling factors occurring at once and so many things depend on one another or affect each other, I had to simply admit, "Yes." Insulin and glucagon are the two opposing hormones that keep blood sugar either increasing or decreasing to normal levels. If we need more glucose, glucagon is produced and through all the complex machinations discussed, we end up losing fat. When there is excess glucose, insulin is produced to bring blood sugar down and part or most of it is stored as fat. We're either storing or retrieving. When carbs are eaten in the smaller and appropriate amounts, in your personal Rx, insulin is held at bay and glucagon is present more often and in higher amounts and voila: body fat loss. An oversimplified explanation, but it is the "whole key."

(Figure 4:7) Work with Your Body

Glucagon ◄──────────────────► Insulin	
• Released when blood sugar is low	• Released when blood sugar too high
• Signals body fat cells to release triglycerides	• Signals body fat cells to convert glucose to fat
• Liver converts fat to glucose	• Signals liver/muscle to store glucose
• Blood/liver/muscle glucose/ glycogen stabilizes	• Causes rebound blood sugar drop
• Hunger decreases	• Hunger increases
• Energy increases	• Energy decreases
• Metabolism increases if protein intake high enough (at least short-term)	

Meal Combinations

The glycemic index is extremely important to your dieting success. Some "nutritionists" don't place much value on this tool, and some act like it doesn't even exist. Yet it can be your greatest asset or your greatest enemy. Many individuals have enjoyed early dieting success with faultless nutrition and then have unknowingly eaten a high-glycemic carb only to be slammed with raging hunger and an insulin-induced tailspin. I think we've all been there – four or five days into a "diet," we find ourselves at the bottom of a gallon of ice cream or lying on the couch with our pants unsnapped after an extended visit to the all-you-can-eat buffet! Now that we know what causes that behavior, we won't let it happen again. The same thing can occur, though, if we go too low on carbohydrates for too long. Anyone who has followed their peers over the low-carb diet cliff knows that powerful hormonal cravings are unleashed that even the strongest-willed can't withstand. Both missteps lead to the same demise. A badly-timed high-glycemic carb or going too long without carbohydrates can lead to low enough blood sugar levels that you suffer with unnecessary hunger, an energy crash, or a head-first dive into a binge.

(Figure 4:8) **Sample Glycemic Index Selections**

The glycemic index essentially rates the speed of digestion of carbohydrates and thus the impact on blood sugar elevation. A zero rating could indicate no carbohydrates present, glucose is rated at a value of 100, and very simple carbohydrates can reach a value much higher than 100.

	Glycemic Index Value	Serving Size	Grams of Carbs per Serving
CEREALS AND BREADS			
All Bran®	30	1/2 cup	15
Oatmeal (rolled oats)	42	1/2 cup (dry)	27
Oatbran bread	47	1 slice	18
Rye bread	58	1 slice	14
Raisin Bran™	61	1/2 cup	19
Pancakes	67	2- 4"	58
Special K™	69	1 cup	21
Bagel, white	72	1	70
Grape Nuts™	75	1/4 cup	22
Shredded Wheat™	75	1 cup	30
English muffin	77	1	14
Whole wheat bread	77	1 slice	12
White bread	80	1 slice	14
Crispix™	87	1 cup	25
Rice Krispies™	87	1 cup	21
Corn Flakes™	92	1 cup	26
SNACKS			
Potato chips	57	2 oz	18
Blueberry muffin	59	3.5 oz	47
Tortilla chips	63	2 oz	30
MET-Rx Bar®	74	3.6 oz	50
Soda crackers	74	5	15
Rice cake	82	1	7
Pretzels	83	1 oz	20

	Glycemic Index Value	Serving Size	Grams of Carbs per Serving
COMMON "STARCH" SOURCES FOR MEALS			
Pasta, wheat	32	1 cup	32
Pasta, white	38	1 cup	32
Sweet potato	44	5 oz	25
Rice, brown	50	1/2 cup	17
Rice, long-grain	61	1/2 cup	18
Rice, white	87	1/2 cup	28
Potato, baked	85	5 oz	30
FRUIT			
Cherries	22	1/2 cup	10
Grapefruit	25	1/2	11
Apple	38	4 oz	15
Pear	38	4 oz	11
Orange	42	4 oz	11
Peach	42	4 oz	11
Grapes	46	1 cup	24
Banana	52	4 oz	24
Raisins	64	1/2 cup	44
Cantaloupe	65	4 oz	6
Pineapple	66	4 oz	10
Watermelon	72	4 oz	6
VEGETABLES			
Broccoli	15	1 cup	5
Cauliflower	15	1 cup	5
Lettuce	15	1 cup	2
Carrots	47	1 cup	10
Peas	48	1/2 cup	10
Corn	60	1/2 cup	18

(The New Glucose Revolution, by Jennie Brand-Miller is recommended for further values and understanding of the glycemic index.)

(Figure 4:9) Sugar Saving Substitutions

Several sugar substitutes exist and may be used to replace sugar sources in cooking, baking, and general sweetening. Though tastes are individual, most artificial sweetener packets can replace two teaspoons of sugar. Non-calorie sweeteners include stevia, aspartame (Equal®), saccharin (Sweet 'N Low®), acesulfame K, and sucralose (Splenda®). My recommendation is stevia, an almost non-caloric sweetening agent derived from a cactus-like plant.

Sugar	Substitutes (packets)	Substitutes (bulk)
2 teaspoons	1 packet	1/2 teaspoon
1/4 cup	6 packets	3 teaspoons
1/3 cup	8 packets	4 teaspoons
1/2 cup	12 packets	6 teaspoons
3/4 cup	18 packets	9 teaspoons
1 cup	24 packets	12 teaspoons

Your own gastrointestinal system actually gives you a carbohydrate safety net, if you know how to use it properly. So far, I've given examples of low- and high-glycemic carb digestive pathways. The glycemic index is a continuum, however, and every food fits in somewhere. Obviously, staying as low as possible will offer the best results with the least "discomfort," but what if you really want a carb source that's not as low on the index as you wish it was? Protein and fat molecules are larger and denser than carbohydrates, and digesting them takes between one and three hours, sometimes longer. The valve (pyloric sphincter) between the stomach and small intestine will stay closed as digestion takes place, opening only one to three times per minute while the food is broken down. If you eat a carb source in combination with fat and protein, the carbohydrate gets caught up in the slowed digestive process. In short, a carb eaten alone will be digested and absorbed much faster than one eaten with fat and protein. Remember, slowed absorption of our carbs is a very good thing! Keep in mind that I want to emphasize the practical side of nutrition as well. Don't misunderstand and think that every meal or snack has to have a "perfect" balance of nutrients or that you can never eat a carbohydrate food alone. Between meals that contain good amounts of protein, sometimes a stand-alone carb is a great snack especially something healthy and low-glycemic like a piece of fruit or vegetables.

CHAPTER FOUR KEY POINTS

1) Carbohydrates provide your body's primary source of energy. Limiting carbohydrates forces the body to use an alternative energy source: body fat.

2) High-glycemic carbs promote body fat creation, increased hunger, and decreased energy.

3) Low-glycemic carbs increase energy, decrease hunger, and help to avoid body fat storage as opposed to high-glycemic carbs.

4) Combining carbs with fat and protein further slows absorption of carbohydrates (refer to later chapter on Meal Planning).

Chapter Five

FAT

The Great Myth

"Eat anything you want as long as you don't eat fat." Have you heard people say such a thing? This has been an accepted "fact" for a long time – until recently that is. You will still find these ideas printed in nutrition textbooks, but we're two fad-diet-generations beyond counting fat grams alone. We've gone from stomping every drop of fat from a chicken breast to painstakingly portioning every bite of food into a perfect balance to eating bacon, burgers, and butter, and now it's time to explain which end is up in all of this mayhem. You now know that carbohydrates are physiologically and practically the most important component in fat loss. But dietary fat comes in a close second and actually works hand-in-hand with carbs. As a matter of fact, a physiology professor of mine was fond of the saying, "Fat is burned in the flames of carbohydrates." You have to have a certain amount of carbohydrates to keep your metabolism normal so you can actually burn body fat. The metabolism of fat, though, comes with even more misconceptions and misinformation. Fat and carbohydrate intake and their effect on weight loss are very intertwined.

There are two main divisions of dietary fat: saturated and unsaturated. Saturated fats most commonly come from animal sources. Beef, pork, dairy products, eggs, and poultry contain saturated fats. Products made with these animal fats – such as butter, cream, and many others – are also saturated. Some choices obviously have a great deal more or less fat than others. For example, fish, chicken, and turkey breast have dramatically less than does beef.

The problems with saturated fats lie primarily in their structure. They are much larger and more stable than unsaturated fats and therefore much harder to break down. Since they don't break down easily, they circulate in the blood stream longer, create higher blood cholesterol levels, lead to atherosclerosis, and much of it ends up being stored as body fat. There really aren't many positive things to say about saturated fats. You've undoubtedly heard the term "trans-fat." A fat can be classified either as a cis- or a trans-fat depending on its chemical structure. Trans-fats in general are those that are solid at room temperature and used in junk food and cheap food processing. Your cell membranes are made up of fat molecules that create receptor sites, like "ports," for certain chemicals like glucose, to be shuttled inside the cell. Trans-fats are rotated and stuck in a "backward" position that doesn't allow this to happen, so the cell can't function properly. Trans-fats have been linked to cancer as well as heart disease (as with any saturated fat).

Unsaturated fats are found mainly in plant sources such as olive oil, canola oil, flaxseed oil, grapeseed oil, borage oil, some nuts, and actually in some fish like salmon. Molecularly, unsaturated fats are smaller, less stable, and easier to break down. Surprisingly, unsaturated fats actually have some important health benefits and can help you lose body fat! Many unsaturated fats contain certain specific "essential fatty acids." Each essential fatty acid has unique properties and benefits to the human body. (Notice they're called "essential," a biological term meaning your body can't produce them so you need to supply them.)

Good Fat?

Most people have heard the terms "good fat" and "bad fat." I can assure you that without some unsaturated dietary fat, body fat loss will be slow at first, minimal at best, and ultimately counterproductive. Let me explain these claims. Some essential fatty acids are the building blocks for certain hormones that control fat loss and storage and the potential for muscle gain and loss. Reread that sentence. One more time, please … Yes, your body produces specific hormones that control how much body fat you can lose or gain and how much muscle you can gain or lose. Your body needs unsaturated fats (essential fatty acids) to create many of these hormones such as testosterone. In a matter of weeks, people who consume a no- or low-fat diet start producing less and less of the "good" hormones that promote body fat loss and muscle gain. Conversely, people who consume 20 to 30% of their calories from unsaturated fat start producing more of these hormones, often above normal levels. With an increase in your hormonal base, you can actually burn more body fat than normal and build more muscle than normal. Research has demonstrated these incredibly positive blood chemistry changes can lead to decreased cholesterol and increased athletic performance. A little of the <u>right</u> dietary fat goes a long way.

(Figure 5:1) Hormones

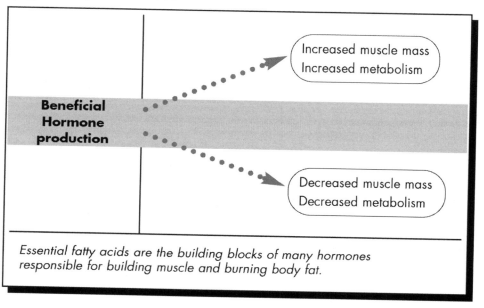

Essential fatty acids are the building blocks of many hormones responsible for building muscle and burning body fat.

I have personally witnessed dramatic decreases in cholesterol and LDL's (low-density lipoproteins, or "bad fat" in the bloodstream) by increasing total dietary fat. I have to qualify this, however, with what I see as a very practical aspect of body fat loss and dieting. Most people who are over weight and eating a poor diet often consume too much refined carbohydrate and too much saturated fat. A few hold-overs from the low-fat craze are eating healthy and fall into the category of "need more good fat," but most of us – whether we care to admit it or not – are killing ourselves on both ends. Therefore, switching to 20 to 30% of calories coming from good fat may cause an overall reduction in body fat. You achieve the best health and best results by eliminating saturated fats and increasing unsaturated fats while keeping carbs in check. You can't leave out carbohydrate control when discussing cholesterol.

Up to 80% of your body's cholesterol is produced in your liver as a result of sugar and runaway insulin. Recall from chapter four that excess carbohydrates result in a conversion to cholesterol and fat. By recommending higher intake of unsaturated fats while controlling carbohydrate levels, I have watched hypercholesterolemic clients (those whose livers produce a significantly larger amount of cholesterol) lower their cholesterol levels and manage them so well that, under the supervision of their physicians, they have been able to eliminate the use of cholesterol-reducing medications. A patient referred to me decreased his blood triglycerides from over 900 to 90 in 3 months using the *Metabolic Transformation* program along with weight training and cardiovascular exercise. A triglyceride level of 900! His poor heart was pumping pudding, not blood! Diet should be the cornerstone of any cholesterol management program, not an afterthought. If you need medication, then take it; heart disease is serious business. However, cholesterol-lowering medication shouldn't be viewed as the cure or an excuse to not lose weight and exercise.

(Figure 5:2) Good Fats/Bad Fats

Unsaturated Fats:	Saturated Fats:
*Easily used as energy	*Difficult to breakdown
*Decrease cholesterol	*Increase cholesterol
*Contain essential fatty acids	
*Necessary for many regenerative body processes	
*Necessary to create certain hormones for optimal health, building muscle, and burning body fat	

Another practical example of the power of correct nutrition is seen in elite athletes whose body composition changes are easily measured and observed. I have personally consulted with and supervised the nutrition of hundreds of bodybuilders preparing for competition. They often need to lose between 15 and 40 pounds of body fat for the contest without losing much muscle, and this can certainly be achieved. However, I have also tested the body composition of competitors who were not receiving proper nutritional support, and I have been amazed at how much muscle can be lost during dieting; quite a contrast to physiologically sound nutrition.

Burgers and Oils

Consciously switching from saturated to unsaturated fat is a lot easier on paper than it is in real life. You can switch from a hamburger to a chicken breast or from three whole eggs to six egg whites, but how are you going to get the good fat into your day? The most practical and healthy ways will be to add certain oils to your food. Over time you will naturally start making better food choices and become more creative. For example, if you have a bowl of oatmeal, add one half to a whole tablespoon of flaxseed oil after it's cooked. Do the same thing with brown rice, yogurt, protein shakes, or anything else that can withstand oil without destroying the taste of the food.

If you're making an egg white omelet, cook it with olive or grapeseed oil instead of a spray. If salad dressing is an area from which you get some of your fat intake, use an Italian dressing made with olive oil instead of a cream-based dressing with saturated fat. Almonds are a very healthy fat source that is very practical for a snack. Watch your serving size; one can is not a serving. Be patient and make the process fun, not overwhelming.

I'm tempted to just leave it at avoiding saturated fat; that would be easier. Adding good fat can be another detail that complicates the process, but essential fatty acids must be integrated into your diet for all of the reasons discussed above. They are necessary for your long-term health, for reducing cholesterol, and for creating hormones. Furthermore, a well-placed snack that contains these concentrated healthy fats will sustain energy and decrease hunger longer.

A Little More Detail

A point that must be understood is how dynamic fat is in the body. If you gained 10 pounds last year, you're not retaining the exact same 10 pounds of body fat that was originally stored. Your body is constantly storing triglycerides in adipose (fat) cells and also releasing them as you need more energy between meals. In fact, adipose cells always store fat after meals and then release it when needed. Fat is actually used for up to 60% of the body's energy needs at rest   A surprising point to most is how easily your body stores dietary fat as body fat. Dietary fat is the easiest nutrient for your body to store as body fat, which makes sense when you think about it. As digested dietary fat is carried past adipose cells in the bloodstream through capillaries, adipose cells simply intake the fat to be stored. As a matter of fact, when you eat just 3% more calories than your body needs at one time, dietary fat is going to be stored in this manner. It takes 25% more food than your body needs at one time to start converting excess carbohydrates into body fat. I know that may sound contradictory as I have made such a big deal of carbohydrates, but don't throw the baby out with the bath water. It is a fact that dietary fat is easier to store as body fat than carbohydrates when calorie intake is more than your body can digest and use at that particular meal. Carbohydrate sources have to be digested, converted into smaller saccharides, dismantled, and then reassembled into fatty acid chains in order to be converted to storable body fat. You need to keep carbs lower and in control to get to the exceptionally accelerated fat loss potential described in chapter one, but you have to keep everything in perspective. Food volume (The Diet Doc Rx) is step one, meal spacing is step two, carb quality and quantity is step three, and then fat closely follows in importance.

If you're tracking this data carefully, you'll see why I stated that overall calorie intake is still always the first step. Total calorie consumption is taken care of by eating within the boundaries of your personal macronutrient range. If you're taking in a moderate amount of fat, even unsaturated fats, a great deal of it can end up stored as fat if carbs and/or overall calories are too high. (Remember the 3% rule from the last paragraph.) However, if your overall calorie intake is

Metabolic Transformation in Action

What a blessing it's been to learn about life-changing nutrition from Joe Klemczewski! There aren't enough superlatives to describe him and his vast knowledge of nutrition and the human body. He genuinely cares about teaching people how to eat so our bodies can be as strong and healthy as God created them to be.

I had been active all my life in many different sports. I excelled in dance (mainly ballet), swimming, aerobics, and karate. I never had to worry about what or how much I ate. It did not affect my weight.

In 1992 my food habits changed. I was eating out a lot and eating more of everything, especially sweets. I had moved to a new city and most of my athletic activities stopped. I jumped five sizes as my weight climbed. I had to do something. I altered what I was eating and started riding my bike and walking. Unfortunately, it wasn't working. My weight increased even more.

For a Christmas gift in 1999 my daughters gave me a gift certificate to Joe's gym. He suggested an appointment to talk about nutrition. Joe taught me that the body needs certain amounts of protein, carbohydrates, and good fat. I also learned I needed to eat six or seven times a day, maintaining these certain amounts that he suggested based on my body size and activity level. I wish anyone with a weight issue could learn what I did from Joe. The results will be good health and body leanness that can be enjoyed for the rest of life.

Because I followed Joe's plan, I immediately started losing weight. In just three months my weight was back where I wanted it. I was gaining muscle and had more energy. I was getting stronger and it felt great. With the weight under control and a commitment to continue exercising, I was able to maintain this accomplishment.

Looking back at those first days in the gym, I was so self-conscious of my legs rubbing together I would wear sweats to hide my legs and, yes, a tee shirt to hide the flab on my arms. Once I lost the weight I timidly wore workout shorts and a workout top in the gym. Someone said, "Tootie, where have you been hiding those muscles?!" Wow! What a mental boost! I felt like I had really accomplished something. That was the end of the cover-me-up clothes! It was the turning point in my training.

Joe made me feel like I was the only client he had. Taking a genuine interest in people, their accomplishments, and helping them achieve their goals, Joe is right there to take you to your maximum potential. After being

continued ⟶

Metabolic Transformation in Action

exposed to some people in the gym and watching how hard they work to compete in bodybuilding and admiring their chiseled bodies, I set a never-before-imagined goal of doing the same.

This was something that I would love to have done in my twenties. Was it possible to do now at age 61? After talking to Joe, it was agreed. I would compete in the 2001 INBF Mid-America Muscle Classic Women's Grand Masters.

I was excited, a little nervous (actually petrified describes it best), but definitely determined. My training became more intense as did my determination. Besides lifting weights, we put a lot of time into selecting music, choreographing a routine, and practicing posing. I learned that behind every bodybuilder on stage there is a great, dedicated team. I had the very best. The encouragement of Joe, his staff, and even their families is awesome and contagious.

It has been amazing to learn from Joe that many of the nutrition ideas I thought to be factual were actually misconceptions that were working against me. I'm thankful Joe has been dedicated to putting his knowledge down on paper. His nutrition manual is the only one in my home. I put it to the test. It worked. Now I'm a 65-year-old woman with a body better than some 20-year-olds. That's proof enough for me.

Share your ultimate goal with Joe, have the right attitude and determination, and he'll see that you achieve it. He encourages you beyond what you think your body is capable. I have complete faith and trust in Joe.

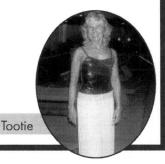

Tootie

lower than your metabolic rate requires, you'll end up using that dietary fat as well as stored fat between meals.

So, if so much of dietary fat ends up being stored as body fat, why not just eliminate it completely? Recall that essential fatty acids play a role in hormone production as well as cellular repair, immune function, and many other life processes. If one is deficient in these essential fatty acids, health consequences cumulatively add physical stress to the body. Another key reason is the focus on keeping blood sugar moderated. Fat takes longer to digest and slows the digestion and assimilation of carbohydrates, so insulin spiking is less of a problem. This type of fat intake has merit, but only if the percentages are representative of an overall calorie intake that's low enough to cause a caloric deficit. As already discussed in detail, the relationship between fats and carbohydrates is very important. If fat intake, for example, is 25% of the total calories instead of 15%, a little lower carbohydrate intake will be necessary to accommodate the additional dietary fat. However, lowering the carbohydrates may then make the practicality of food intake difficult, and energy levels may drop. Thus, a slightly lower fat intake, allowing for more carbohydrates, may be necessary. Some flexibility between carbohydrates and fat is allowed in the Diet Doc Rx and you should

(Figure 5:3) Saturated Fat Reducing Tips

1) Use non-stick cooking spray to reduce fat or use unsaturated oils to increase "good" fat when cooking.
2) Boil, roast, bake, or steam food in place of frying.
3) Use egg whites in place of whole eggs when baking. Two egg whites equal one whole egg.
4) Use skim milk in place of whole or 2% milk.
5) Choose low- or no-fat yogurts, mayo, and salad dressings.
6) Use spices and fat-free condiments such as salsa to spice up food.
7) Use applesauce in place of butter and/or oil in baked goods.
8) Make sure canned tuna, chicken, and other meats are packed in water, not oil.
9) Choose the leanest cuts of meat.
10) Trim fat from meat.

feel comfortable trying different combinations as long as you stay within both ranges.

A discussion of fat intake and dietary theory wouldn't be complete without commenting on the ketogenic (low-carb) camp. What do we do with the "experts" that would have us eat unlimited amounts of fat and protein but eschew carbs with the promise of a lean, muscular physique? Since excess carbs are easily converted to body fat and lead to insulin-induced lethargy, higher risk of diabetes and heart disease, and many other health perils, it's correct applied knowledge to control carbs and their quality. It's also imperative to make sure that carbs are low enough to not supply all the energy requirements of the body.

AVERAGE JOE PHYSIOLOGY

Avoid Fat Altogether?

The question of which is worse – excess dietary fat or excess carbohydrates in relation to cardiovascular disease – is still largely misunderstood. Even if you're only 20 years old, this is a concept to understand completely. Coronary artery blockage often invokes the imagery of some fatty deposits that can be scoured away with proper eating and exercise at will. The truth is that the atherosclerotic fat that collects on the artery walls starts a process that isn't entirely reversible. The plaque that forms creates an inflammatory condition by which collagen also collects, creating a fibrous lesion. Even as plaque and cholesterol are reduced through diet and exercise, some narrowing of the vessels remain permanent. The answer is to be responsible and heart-healthy early in life and maintain it.

The average American diet includes 40% of calories from fat. Though 20 to 30% is more appropriate, that still leaves a large amount of calories that one can actively choose from unsaturated, natural sources, or from saturated and trans-fatty acids. Obviously the latter will perpetuate the process of heart disease but many choose another avenue of proactive dieting. Some are swayed to decrease overall fat consumption as low as possible and eat more carbohydrates to replace those calories. Studies show that type of dieting can lower LDL-cholesterol levels, but it also tends to lower "good" HDL-cholesterol levels and can increase triglyceride levels. When replacing carbohydrates with monounsaturated natural oils, studies show a decrease in triglycerides and an increase in HDL's. Polyunsaturated oils did decrease LDL's but didn't have much of an effect on HDL's or triglycerides. For heart health, the best combination is to keep carbohydrates low enough so that saturated fats can be replaced by some monounsaturated fats. (Olive oil and almonds are two of the richest sources of monounsaturated fats.)

A high-carb diet in which protein and fat intake is low will not allow for much body fat loss because the body will have little reason to access a secondary energy source such as body fat. If you take the opposite extreme and eliminate almost all carbohydrates from the body, then stored fat will be released at a very rapid rate. Though seemingly used successfully by many bodybuilders, this type of dieting has its problems. First, adipose cells release fat to be used as energy in the form of glycerol and fatty acids. Body cells intake the glycerol and fatty acids to metabolize them into energy through the Kreb's cycle, but glucose fragments <u>must</u> be present. (Hmm…looks like my physiology professor was right, fat is burned in the flames of carbohydrates.) Let me repeat this: glucose fragments (carbs) must be present to burn body fat for energy through the very efficient Kreb's cycle within every cell; but it isn't the only way. If glucose isn't available, fatty acids can combine with each other to form ketone bodies that can also be used by most cells for energy conversion. The rate of body fat usage for energy can be great using this method of diet, but the problems with this mechanism are many.

(Figure 5:4) The Dynamic Nature of Energy

- Blood sugar too low
- Glucagon released
- Glycogen harvested
- Fat released

- Blood sugar too high
- Insulin released
- Glycogen stored
- Fat stored

Body Fat Cell

- Dietary fat in blood stream, when carbs are normal or high, gets stored easily as fat.
- Dietary fat in blood stream, when carbs are low, gets converted and used as glucose in the place of stored body fat.

Ketogenic dieting may be effective only if fat intake isn't too excessive. Remember, adipose cells are just waiting to suck in new fat to store after meals. One of the two greatest problems of low-carb dieting is that carbs are the most protein-sparing nutrient we eat. If carbs are too low for too long, you'll lose muscle no matter how much protein you eat, period! Secondly, the brain and nervous system prefer glucose, not ketone bodies, for energy. Low energy and inefficient nervous system activity leave workouts low-key, weak, and less effective – not to mention fatigue in daily life. If you enjoy feeling lousy, having no energy, craving carbohydrates intensely, and being prone to binging, then low-carb dieting is for you. Ketogenic dieting certainly allows you to burn more fat initially because of the immense carb deficit, but increasing fat intake too much can cause a great deal of fat storage. Two steps forward, two steps back. The few who have successfully employed this type of dieting leave me wondering how much easier it would have been had they dieted "correctly" in the first place.

So, what's the take-home message about fat? If you're in a maintaining, isocaloric stage of non-dieting, you can successfully eat 30% or more of your calories from fat sources without a problem – though I would chose approximately 20% of your total so that more protein and/or carbs can be consumed. The key is in the word "isocaloric," or eating the same amount of total calories that your body uses for energy, so that whatever ratios you chose, you won't store new body fat. If you're dieting to a very low level, you can save yourself from taking too many steps backward by cutting fat intake to 10 to 15% of total calories. This simply means less fat will be available for storage after meals and the amount of stored fat used between meals for energy will be coming from a faster-shrinking supply. I wouldn't recommend staying too low for too long, though, as you may trigger the metabolic ill effects of too low a fat intake. Carbohydrate control and planning are just as important as dietary fat, but in reality the two go hand-in-hand. Many people who obsess about carbs alone end up snacking on too many nuts, extra peanut butter, and other high-fat, low-carb foods, only to increase direct fat storage from the increased fat intake. When taking in a limited amount of fat, be sure to make the most of what you get and supplement with essential fatty acids. Don't lose sight of the big picture: dietary fat intake is a critical part of your success, but it has to be just one piece of a comprehensive plan to work!

One last word about fats: have a steak once in awhile. A small percentage of saturated fat isn't going to throw you into cardiac arrest, and if your cholesterol is actually too low, you can suffer from low energy, low hormonal levels, and even depression. This is admittedly a low population, but does happen, especially with those who are very disciplined and deep into a weight-loss cycle.

CHAPTER FIVE KEY POINTS

• • • •➤ 1) Saturated fats are found primarily in animal sources.

• • • •➤ 2) Saturated fats lead to heart disease and body fat.

• • • •➤ 3) Unsaturated fats contain essential fatty acids that are necessary for many body processes.

• • • •➤ 4) Unsaturated fats in the right amounts are necessary to lose the maximal amount of body fat and to build muscle.

Chapter Six

PROTEIN

So Many Choices!

Just as most saturated fats come from animal sources, so does protein. Houston, we have a problem. We need protein, but we don't want saturated fat. Fish, chicken and turkey breast, ostrich, egg whites, and even soy-based meat substitutes offer an alternative to foods high in saturated fat like beef, pork, dairy products, and whole eggs. These healthier foods are now commonly found on the menus of most restaurants making it easier to obtain on the go.

Another convenient protein choice comes in the form of protein powders, shakes, and bars. The reason professional athletes endorse supplement companies (besides getting paid) is that they actually use their products. It can be a lot easier to get supplemental protein in the form of a great tasting shake or bar, especially in on-the-run situations. I couldn't eat properly and still see a high volume of patients and clients without an occasional bar or shake to supplement our whole-food meals. Getting some of your protein from sources like shakes and bars will also help you avoid feeling like you're growing a beak from eating so much poultry!

Why Protein?

Most bodybuilders would correctly tell you that you need protein to build muscle. They would probably also tell you, however, that you need two to three times what you really require. If you asked a vegetarian about protein, you might learn how to make a dozen eggs last for a year. Your body has the ability to survive either extreme, but you will pay the price for each. You can survive without much protein at all, but you will strip the muscle right off your bones and impair your ability to build the healthiest cells. Too much protein, as advocated by some muscle magazines (owned by protein supplement companies), and you

Metabolic Transformation in Action

You've probably heard a lot of successful dieters say, "If I can lose weight on this diet, anyone can!" But in the case of Dr. Joe's plan, it really is true!

I had all the normal "excuses" for not being able to lose weight. I was over 40, had an autoimmune disorder that affected my joints, many other medical conditions, and a "sluggish" metabolism. Some doctors even suggested I just be satisfied with maintaining my current weight. But at 5'4" and 260 pounds, my blood pressure, blood sugar, and cholesterol were at life-threatening levels. I started on a diet program from a popular diet book and made some progress. It wasn't specific enough to help me when I "got stuck." I started regaining the weight without any idea how to reverse it. By June 2003 I was completely convinced that no diet would ever help me.

I called Dr. Joe, we decided to meet, and the rest is "history."

As of October 2005, I have lost over 120 pounds and am close to my goal – weighing 130 pounds after losing 130 pounds. My latest cholesterol test (non-fasting) was 178, compared to totals in the 220's before. My blood sugar is within normal levels and I hope to be free of all blood pressure medicines in the next few months. My joint problems have all but disappeared, along with my other health problems. No one recognizes the "old me" and I have no intention of going back there.

So what makes his diet and exercise plan different? For one thing, you don't start eating special foods that help you lose weight as long as you're on them – but let you regain your weight once you return to normal eating. You start by gaining an awareness of the protein, fat, and carbohydrate balances in the foods you currently eat. It was a huge wakeup call for me – mainly the carbohydrates. I had no idea I was eating so many carbs in a day. Just understanding that problem started me down the road to better eating. Dr. Joe wants you to understand the importance of looking at the foods you normally eat. I was able to look for the foods I liked, find out how to moderate them, or substitute them, and design my own plan for diet success. I put the counts of the foods I normally ate into an Excel spreadsheet. I still carried the "food count" book with me so I could calculate the values for new foods. If you can control the portions and fit the counts into your daily diet, no food is completely off limits. Joe's plan lets you take ownership of your own diet plan. With my busy schedule, I frequently ate in restaurants and have still been successful with the diet.

continued ⟶

Metabolic Transformation in Action

He also helped me understand the importance of not only aerobic but also strength exercises and has helped guide me to an effective training program. I'm still "perfecting" that part! I am not a bodybuilder or an athletic person – I have trouble with coordination (walking and chewing gum!). I always thought my lack of skills would hamper my effectiveness with exercise. Not true.

I'm still not coordinated, I'm still not a bodybuilder, but I am getting to be a thinner, fitter person thanks to this plan. I'm a normal, everyday person. Believe me, if I can do it, so can you!

Does the plan work? You can probably tell from my "before" and "after" photos the answer is yes! All I can say is I used to be a size 22 and now I'm a size 4. How many 46-year-olds weigh what they did at age 18 after spending years and years well over 200 pounds? It's safe to say that reading his book and following his advice has changed my life forever. He has given me the specific tools to keep this up and to help myself recover from those inevitable "holiday" relapses!

I can't thank him enough. But I can encourage all of you – it's never too late and you can do it!

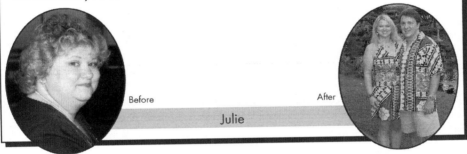

Before
After
Julie

may spend a lifetime in a state of acidosis creating a host of degenerative diseases. Others warn you could end up on the kidney transplant waiting list. So, how much is best? Kind of an important question, don't you think?

The amounts of protein I advocate are designed to abundantly meet the body's requirements without the risk of undesirable effects. Protein is very important in creating new cells, such as red blood cells, skin cells, liver cells, etc., as well as in the maintenance and metabolic activities of every system in your body. If protein intake is too low, your entire body eventually suffers, even your immune system. At first, you can withstand protein depletion very efficiently because you have so much stored. Protein is broken down into amino acids, which are used in just about every chemical reaction that takes place within your body. Amino acids are made up of nitrogen compounds that circulate in your

(Figure 6:1) Protein Utilization

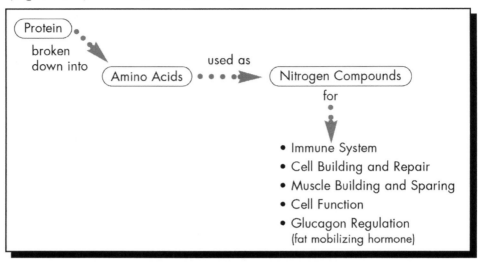

bloodstream and are stored in a few places, mostly as skeletal muscle and some in the liver. So yes, you can live a long time without protein, and even longer with insufficient amounts of protein; your body will simply break down your muscle tissue to provide what it needs. It's a great survival mechanism, but as far as I'm concerned, I don't want to knowingly lose any muscle and neither should you.

I estimate protein requirements for active people. If you aren't performing rigorous exercise at least three to four times per week, choose the lower end of suggested protein ranges shown in chapter two. If you train extremely hard or perform several sessions of cardiovascular work per week, you may actually need to go slightly above the suggested amount.

Variety is the Spice of Life

Every protein has a specific amino acid profile. This means each protein source may be higher or lower in certain amino acids than other protein sources. There are many rating scales that attempt to build a hierarchy among protein sources by assigning values and deeming them "high-" or "low-quality" protein sources. There is merit to these types of ratings. However, even the highest-rated protein source is low in certain amino acids, and vice versa.

Vegetarians may have also heard that you have to combine certain foods to "make a complete protein." You're covered on this principle on two different fronts. First, digestion, absorption, and circulation keep the amino acids that you consume available for hours, and they can be augmented with other amino acids in previous or later meals. The liver also stores a small reserve of amino acids that it uses when necessary. While we're on the subject of protein and vegetarianism, I want to make sure you understand you can succeed without animal protein. I still recommend getting at least the minimal suggested protein intake in your Diet Doc Rx for all the reasons discussed above. Think about it: if you avoid protein as a vegetarian, most of your food will come from carbohydrates causing the same physiological and behavioral challenges to health and weight loss. I have had many vegetarian clients lose weight, drop their cholesterol, and regain surprising energy by trimming starch and adding a couple protein shakes a day or other protein source acceptable to them.

The bottom line, therefore, is simply to enjoy a variety of protein sources throughout your day so that you take in a variety of amino acids. Keep in mind that saturated fats should be kept to a minimum so your diet leaves room for high-quality unsaturated fats and essential fatty acids.

Back to Hormones

Just as carbohydrates can affect your body in a positive or negative way through the modulation of the hormone insulin, protein creates a similar effect through the hormone glucagon. To oversimplify, insulin is released when you eat carbs; glucagon is released when you eat protein. Just as insulin is a storage hormone, glucagon is a retrieval, or mobilizing, hormone. It actually promotes glucose to be used as energy. When glucose isn't present in large enough quantities (because you've been so good at limiting your carbs and sticking to your daily totals!) glucagon helps mobilize body fat to be burned as energy. Hence the importance of breaking your daily macronutrient totals up so that you can have protein in most meals.

Think of insulin and glucagon as representing two opposite metabolic stimuli. Insulin is present, active, and dominant if carbohydrate intake is too high,

AVERAGE JOE PHYSIOLOGY

Why Protein Helps

High-protein, low-carb diets have cycled into the diet fad rotation about every 20 years since the 1950s. Though we can all agree that carbohydrates are a critical – maybe the most important – variable in dieting, it can be taken to an unhealthy and even dangerous level. Many of these diets allow unlimited amounts of protein as long as carbs stay ultra-low. Naysayers claim that too high of a protein intake can be stressful to the kidneys, but however logical, very little evidence exists to support kidney damage. Yet there are other reasons to avoid this extreme approach.

First, studies show a very high incidence of weight regain, often with decreased lean body mass. Eliminating carbohydrates will reduce blood levels of insulin – a very good thing – but to such a low level that your body becomes very insulin sensitive. A significant hormone, adipsin, works inside the body fat cell to help regulate how much blood glucose will get pulled into the cell to be stored as fat. Its activation is modulated by insulin. Since ketogenic metabolism is less efficient than glucose metabolism, the body becomes more sensitive to glucose as it desperately wants to use it for energy. When in this hyper-sensitive state, the hormone adipsin has been measured to be many times more effective at storing glucose as body fat. This is the basis of the "starvation-mode" cliché often used as an excuse for not losing weight. The truth is, one has to be consuming virtually no carbohydrates for approximately eight weeks to have an appreciable change, but if one remains on a very-low carb diet, adipsin sensitivity will happen. The body literally becomes a fat-storing machine. The process will reverse itself as carbohydrate intake increases, but in the meantime, much body fat may be regained.

The second most important reason to avoid low-carb diets is the negative effect they have on mood and brain function. The brain cannot use free fatty acids for energy, has very little amounts of glycogen stores, and consumes a whopping 20% of the body's total energy at rest. It can use ketone bodies as energy in a fasting state, but mental function is greatly compromised. Eating moderate carbs is a prescription for success as well as for a sharp noodle!

and your body is thus in a storage mode. Glucagon is present, active, and dominant when carbohydrate intake is lower and protein intake is higher, thus promoting fat mobilization. Glucagon is one of several hormones that can "unlock" body fat cells and is the most powerful that is nutrition-dependent. Others are more exercise-dependent. When you combine the most effective nutrition and exercise to maximize these hormones, you truly are working with your body for the fastest progress.

Protein also has the greatest "thermic potential" among macronutrients. This means that when you eat protein, your metabolism rises because protein digestion requires more energy. Protein is very important for health and body composition. This, along with hormonal considerations such as glucagon, is the reason many new studies are showing that diets higher in protein and lower (notice I say "lower" and not "low") in carbs can cause much faster body fat loss – even with the same amount of calories!

I recommend that if you feel like you need more food on a particular day than your macronutrient range allows, it's better to eat a little more protein than to end up binging. But if you do this too often you'll find overall calories too high and insulin will once again be a factor in keeping you from losing as much weight. Remember that calories (overall energy intake) are always step one.

CHAPTER SIX KEY POINTS

• • • ▶ 1) Protein is found in animal meats and sometimes in small amounts in certain beans and plants.

• • • ▶ 2) Supplemental protein can be found in many types of protein shakes and bars.

• • • ▶ 3) Protein is necessary for many vital processes in the body as well as muscle growth.

• • • ▶ 4) Protein sources have different amino acid profiles, making it advantageous to vary your protein choices.

• • • ▶ 5) Eating protein raises your metabolism, and through the actions of the hormone glucagon, assists you in losing body fat faster.

Chapter Seven

MEAL RATIOS

Better Living through Chemistry

Few authors have ever validated their "diets" with actual research. The reason we have been tossed to and fro, from one diet to another, is that they promise great results; but unfortunately their diets are physiologically unverified. For the average person, nutrition is often a black hole of mystery and marketing. Only recently have scientists started conducting thorough research on food's affect on health and body composition. Hormones, exercise, and food all affect nutritional status. Obviously, the fuel we put in our bodies multiple times a day is the key factor.

Measuring Cups and Calculators

Reviewing a little of what I've discussed already will help to pull this section together. Eating the right amount of food per day (The Diet Doc Rx) and dividing that food into small meals (power spacing) are the first steps in creating your eating structure. Recall the importance of each macronutrient and some of the better choices of each. The big questions, then, are: do I have to have the same amount of protein, carbs, and fat in each meal? And, do I have to have the same ratios of nutrients in each meal?

Yes and no. To allow some flexibility, I suggest a small range in each macronutrient rather than a rigid amount of food per meal or per day. I'll explain my rationale, but first let me offer that once you are locked into a "normal" eating pattern within your daily totals, you will achieve the best results if your meals represent a fairly even distribution of macronutrients throughout the day. Consuming 60 grams of carbs in a meal and 10 in the next just isn't going to cut it. You want a good ratio of nutrients in each meal to promote stable blood sugar levels and therefore stable energy and less hunger.

Metabolic Transformation in Action

I have struggled with my weight since I was in my late 20's after I delivered our daughter, Sarah. Each year I gained a few pounds until at 49 years of age I weighed over 200. Because weight was such an issue in my family growing up, I had sworn off all diets. I didn't really eat a lot of food, but was eating all the wrong foods. But, during all those years, I continued exercising three to five times a week – walking, riding my bike, swimming, tennis, etc. So, for a heavy woman, I was in fairly good shape. Paul, as a farmer, was always very active. He, like me, was gaining a few pounds each year. His doctor told him that he needed to lose weight, especially since his cholesterol was high. In 2003, I was unable to exercise consistently at all. I was student teaching the first half of the year, and beginning a new position at the University of Southern Indiana as a math instructor the second half of the year. I was so busy that I had no time to exercise or to cook. At least two to three times week we went out to eat fast food – cheeseburgers, french fries, and Coke – food I never thought I could live without. Because I wasn't able to exercise, my weight ballooned to 218. By December 2003 I was experiencing a lot of knee pain and shoulder pain. I was also very tired and just sick of living like this. I was finally ready to change my eating habits.

We had heard about Dr. Joe and his eating plan two years prior. I e-mailed him and set up an appointment in January. I knew that if I didn't do it then, I wouldn't feel like it in January. I remember going to that first appointment thinking, "What am I doing? I am still so snowed under from my job, I can't put any effort into this now." But, I also knew that if I didn't do it now, I wouldn't do it later. Paul agreed to go with me, knowing that he needed to lose too. He didn't want to go on any diet, because he was afraid that we would just gain it back. We met with Dr. Joe and he explained the physiology of eating and losing weight. I had told myself that, yes, I needed to lose weight, but, more importantly, I needed to learn how to eat right. Dr. Joe gave us each our plan of right eating – the amount of protein, carbs, and fat we should eat each day and how to put them together. Then he sent us home to implement it. We ate our last fast food dinner and went to bed. We got up the next morning and looked at each other – where do we begin? Dr. Joe had given us a sample menu for one day, but we were totally clueless on the nutritional value of any food. The first few days (and weeks) were difficult as we were struggling to put our foods together and staying under our prescribed amount of protein, carbs, and fat. I started

continued ⟶

Metabolic Transformation in Action

a spreadsheet to help us add up our grams each day. We soon realized that starting at dinner and planning backwards was the key for us. The eating plan allowed us the freedom to eat what we like, within reason. It didn't stop us from eating out or eating with our friends. It just gave us the tools and the information we needed to make our eating healthy, yet, fit our likes.

Every Wednesday morning Paul and I would weigh in front of each other and mark our progress. We still do that to this day. The eating plan worked like clockwork. Each week I lost about one to one and a half pounds and Paul would lose one and a half to two pounds. By the end of May, Paul had lost 50 pounds, meeting his goal of 175. I continued on, losing 75 pounds by the middle of October, and meeting my goal of 145. As I began eating better, I also began training to walk/run the mini-marathon in Indianapolis. By April, I had lost 35 pounds and finished a min-marathon in less than 3 hours. By October, I was down to my goal weight and participated in my second mini-marathon in Evansville and finished in just over two and a half hours. Paul continues farming and working outside each day. We both feel so much better. My knees and shoulders don't hurt anymore. We both have more energy, and love being able to go into any store and buy clothes without trying them on. I used to wear a size 22, but now I wear a size 10. Paul went from a size 38 to a size 34. Our eating plan has become a change of life for us. We will never look on food the same. We don't always eat like we should, but we keep close tabs on our weight and adjust our eating to match. Many people have followed Dr. Joe's plan after seeing what we were able to do.

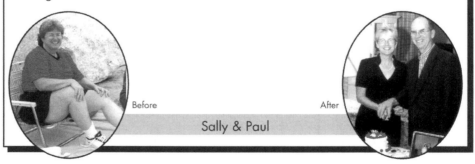

Before

After

Sally & Paul

There are, however, times when some flexibility is not only helpful, but simply the right thing to do. For example, if you've just performed an intense workout, your next meal may include a little higher percentage of carbohydrates to refill the stored glycogen (sugar) used in the muscle tissue. If you're going to bed soon, and you're hungry, it would be better to have a higher percentage of

Okay, So You Can Blame Mom and Dad a Little

Though genetics are often wrongly blamed for weight management woes, it would be a great mistake to dismiss the subject. As much as we have learned about genetics in the last generation, it is a case of "the more you learn; the more you realize you don't know." Two clear issues regarding weight gain genetics are body fat cell volume and hormones that control hunger. We all have a genetic range of body fat cells that we will be born with. The proliferation of these cells is greatest during the first year of life and then a second surge is possible during puberty. It is difficult to actually increase the number of body fat cells at other times except in the case of extreme and rapid weight gain. Most fat storage is done within the number of body fat cells already created. However, this can be a wide range, for example, 15 billion in 1 person or 250 billion in another. The sheer cell mass of the extra fat cells is significant but more of a factor is that fat cells don't remain "empty." Triglycerides can be removed and kept to a minimum but the dynamic activity of metabolism makes it likely that small amounts of reserves will be left. This also increases the body's ability and ease of storing body fat – a major disadvantage. Multiply that by an exponentially large amount of body fat cells and it's easy to see how some people have "bigger frames," have "always been hefty", and have similar genetic shapes compared to parents and siblings. This isn't a life-sentence to be or remain obese, but it certainly makes it more challenging for some.

Leptin is a hormone discovered to control hunger and could be a key component in obesity and potentially a future pharmacological focus on treating it. Body fat cells secret leptin into the bloodstream proportionately to the amount of stored triglycerides. The hormone decreases hunger. This discovery gives credence to the "set point" theory describing that our bodies have a "preferred" weight. If the message isn't being transmitted properly that "there is enough fat stored," a person wouldn't feel satisfied and would continue to eat. This is a very exciting area of study but no one knows the outcome or possible side effects as of yet. Diet and exercise, though, work every time.

protein and less carbs. This will actually stimulate more growth hormone to be released at night and suppress insulin, which inhibits growth hormone. You will also find that you're hungrier during some points of the day than you are at others. You may need a small meal only two hours after eating during the morning, but you can go three hours after lunch. Some meals will be larger, and some smaller. The point is: flexibility is often helpful due to schedules, is often physiologically necessary, and can help with your own compliance to succeed with this new eating pattern. There is a balance, however, between what is right and perfect nutritionally and the level you can achieve in your daily life.

CHAPTER SEVEN KEY POINTS

• • • •➤ 1) Keep nutrient totals spaced throughout meals.

• • • •➤ 2) Allow yourself flexibility when necessary regarding meal ratios but stay within your nutrient totals for the day.

• • • •➤ 3) Remember power spacing!

• • • •➤ 4) Learn your body's natural hunger patterns and adjust meal spacing accordingly, allowing for some flexibility.

Chapter Eight

RECIPES AND FOOD PREPARATION

Just Tell Me What to Eat!

Most new clients sit across from me in full trust, expecting body fat loss and positive health changes similar to what they have seen in the person who referred them. Occasionally, however, clients want to skip all of the teaching and learning and jump right into a template-based diet. A mild version of this request is a client that asks for recipes and meal plans, and then hints at wanting the inclusion of an entire daily menu. The more severe version comes from clients who beg for a written menu to follow, or simply "won't be able to succeed." "I promise, just tell me what to eat and I'll eat it! I don't care if I eat the same thing every meal, every day!"

For this client, I predict failure. This is a client who has tried everything else and has failed more as a result of lacking initiative and discipline than due to a faulty nutrition plan. Sorry to be so blunt, but keep reading – you'll see what I mean. Though it seems easier, you don't want to follow a meal-by-meal plan written by us or anyone else. Nobody knows what foods you like, what your schedule is, or what challenges may be unique to you. You have to learn to interact with food – any food – and put it into your daily plan successfully. For the sake of reference and to start you with some ideas, though, I have provided a small number of meals for you to view as examples. But, our goal is for you to create your own food intake based on the nutritional values proposed in chapter two.

When a client comes to me through a class, a consultation, or my online program, I purposely make the first step personal menu planning. My client goes home and figures out what he or she is going to eat the next day, making the best food choices, keeping nutrient totals and meal spacing as even as possible, and creating four to six meals that fall into their personal Diet Doc Rx. Yes, it takes a food count book, a calculator, an eraser, and a lot of patience. Once you've taken this step, however, you are well on your way to success because you have a framework from which to build a pattern. You will quickly learn to substitute a variety of food and meal choices and stay within your plan. Without this planning, you will likely not be able to continue successfully. The responsibility I ask you to assume is the driving force that makes the nutritional elements work in your daily life. You will learn to adapt, be creative, and begin an ongoing process of cumulative learning. You will become your own best nutritionist. You will succeed.

Yet, many people who join a "weight-loss center" end up gaining back all the lost weight within one year. These chain weight-loss centers pride themselves on making it easy for their customers by giving them diet plans, meal cards, follow-along daily menus, and even prepackaged food. On this issue, I gladly walk in the opposite direction. Studies have determined that the majority of the people who engage in these programs weigh more one year later than the day they walked in the door. The initial ease offered by a menu is quickly complicated by the fact that you have a different schedule, different tastes, different goals, and different metabolic needs than everyone else. Secondly, you learn nothing about nutrition and how to make permanent changes unless you go through a progressive learning process. It's a little more difficult and time consuming on the front end, but the education will stick in your brain and will make it easier for the rest of your life. Your ability to control your weight will forever be greater.

What's That?

Many successful clients have suggested I write a recipe book. Maybe some day I will, but for now I have included a great recipe section for you to get started. Along with the meal samples provided, you now have a great amount of food information to help create innumerable days of good meals within your personal Rx. And, that's what it's all about: using foods you like to merge "natural" eating habits into the ranges that will accomplish your goal. Check out the book store or library for full recipe books that suit your taste and the type of meal ratios you're looking for. There are books that cater to lower-carb meals, lower-fat meals, or whatever you need help with in structuring your menu. Begin with the realization that eating the right foods in the right amounts is your focus. You don't have to make a meal for your family and a separate meal for yourself. Simply take the right foods in the right amounts. This leads to why I devalue recipes slightly. You don't have to have elaborate recipes and exotic ingredients, or even "special" foods, to diet and eat correctly. Right foods, right amounts. I can throw a can of tuna in a bowl with a cup of brown rice, stir in a half a tablespoon of flaxseed oil, pour on some salsa, and I'm ready to eat. Breakfast? No problem! Mix a scoop of strawberry protein powder into my already-cooked half-cup of oatmeal, add some almonds or oil, and I'm off to the office. Creativity! You may get some funny looks once in awhile, but you'll have the last laugh. When you put this book down tonight, take a tour of your kitchen and start looking at the three macronutrient categories on the food labels. Some will pleasantly surprise you, and some will spur you to put green Poison Control Center stickers on the box. Now you're taking an active role in your own nutrition.

Breakfast without Sugar

Most breakfast selections are a disastrous way to start your day. Sugar and refined (high-glycemic) flour are used to create very tasty cereals, as long as you don't mind a little extra body fat, low energy, and hunger. You're not a cereal person? How about a doughnut or a "healthier" refined-flour bagel with 50 grams of carbs? Breakfast bars, pastries – yep, same story.

Breakfast is actually a difficult meal for most people due to time constraints and/or a lack of food ideas. Unless you want my tuna and salsa concoction for breakfast, pay attention. Protein in the morning is difficult unless you plan ahead. Take time to cook egg white combinations or utilize a protein substitute. Scrambled egg whites (with one whole egg – if you like – and the extra fat fits in your meal plan) cooked in olive or canola oil, joined by oat or rye toast, make a great breakfast. You can even get fancy with different omelets.

Oatmeal (watch for added sugar in flavored brands) is an excellent choice and can be fortified with fat and protein, as noted earlier. Meal replacement shakes can also be very helpful. These are protein powders packaged in individual servings (or large canisters) and these products make great shakes in a blender where you can add your choice of high-quality oil and low-glycemic fruit if you chose to "spend" that amount of carbohydrate at breakfast. You can't get much quicker than that.

A thought that may help you decrease your reliance on huge amounts of processed carbs at breakfast is to view it as just another meal. Bodybuilders will sometimes eat yet another chicken breast and green beans for breakfast (I know, I know...they're not normal – I can attest to that!). You don't need to go to that extreme, but who said that we need eight ounces of juice and a stack of pancakes for breakfast? It is an important meal to not skip, but I challenge you to try increasing the protein and decreasing the carbs. You'll be less hungry in the later morning, and you'll have more energy. Plus, you will have saved more carbs for later meals and snacks. It's all good!

Lunch and Supper the Easy Way

Lunch and supper, or even whole food snacks, can easily be pieced together by combining compatible protein, carbohydrate, and fat choices. Choose your protein source and then add complimentary carbs and fat. If it's a chicken breast, decide whether you want pasta, brown rice, a sweet potato – it's your choice. Add a limited amount of a healthy fat source (if necessary to reach your suggested nutrient totals) and eat with confidence. A deli (chicken or turkey breast) sandwich can be made with low-glycemic bread and condiments. Health food stores even have mayonnaise made with canola oil instead of saturated fat. A chicken breast salad with a little Italian dressing is a great choice. The salad vegetables give you great carbs and the dressing gives you olive oil. Your creativity and planning are the only factors that can inhibit you from enjoying great tasting food and easy-to-prepare meals.

(Figure 8:1) Simple Breakfasts

Food Source	Protein	Carbs	Fat
3 egg whites	12	0	0
1 piece whole grain toast	2	13	1
1 tsp. canola oil	0	0	4
(to cook eggs)			
Total	14	13	5
(Great light breakfast that is very balanced and filling.)			
6 egg whites/1 yolk	27	0	6
2 pieces whole grain toast	4	26	2
1 tsp. canola oil	0	0	4
Total	31	26	12
(Similar breakfast but larger.)			
1/2 cup (dry) oats	5	27	3
1 scoop protein powder	30	5	1
1/2 tbsp. flaxseed oil	0	0	6
Total	35	32	10
Mix powder and oil into oats after oats are cooked.			
(Protein powder is optional but does significantly fortify this already great breakfast.)			
1/2 cup low-fat cottage cheese	13	4	5
4 egg whites	16	0	0
1 tsp. canola oil (to cook)	0	0	4
Chopped omelet veggies	0	3	0
Total	29	7	9
Mix cottage cheese and egg whites in bowl, then make omelet.			
(High-protein, low-carb breakfast that is versatile and tastes great.			
Add carb sources such as toast if desired.)			

Food Source	Protein	Carbs	Fat
1/2 cup low-fat, plain yogurt	8	10	2
1 scoop protein powder	30	5	1
1/8 cup almonds	3	3	7
1/4 cup (dry) oats	3	13	1
Totals	44	31	11

Mix everything together into yogurt. May substitute high-fiber cereal for oats.

May add fruit for more carbs if needed.

Cut in half if necessary for your meal plan.

(This quick option tastes like dessert for breakfast!)

Food Source	Protein	Carbs	Fat
Meal replacement shake	40	20	1
1/2 tbsp. flaxseed oil	0	0	5
8 oz. skim milk	8	4	2
Totals	48	24	8

May substitute 1 tbsp. peanut butter for flaxseed oil. May use water instead of milk.

Blend in mixer with ice. May use scoop of protein powder instead of meal

replacement packet to decrease protein and carbs.

(This is a quick but significant jump-start for the day.)

Food Source	Protein	Carbs	Fat
1 cup high-fiber cereal	3	35	1
1 cup skim milk	8	4	2
1/2 scoop protein powder	15	2	1
Totals	26	41	4

Mix vanilla protein powder well in milk, pour on cereal.

(Can't get much faster than this, but measure well; the carbs in cereal add up fast!)

Food Source	Protein	Carbs	Fat
3 egg whites	12	0	0
2 pieces low-fat turkey bacon	6	0	2
1 tsp. canola oil (to cook)	0	0	4
2 pieces whole grain toast	4	26	2
Totals	22	26	8

May use whole grain pancakes instead of toast. May drop 1 piece of toast to

decrease carbs. May make into sandwich.

(If you have time, this is a classic!)

(Figure 8:2) Lunch and Dinner

Food Source	Protein	Carbs	Fat
5 oz. chicken breast	35	0	5
1/2 cup rice	2	22	0
Salad or can of green beans	0	10	0
2 tbsp. low-/no-fat dressing	0	2	2
Totals	37	34	7

(This is a "full-size" lunch or supper that is complete in all categories.)

Food Source	Protein	Carbs	Fat
4 oz. deli turkey breast	28	0	4
2 pieces whole grain bread	4	26	2
Lettuce/tomato	0	0	0
Mustard	0	0	0
Totals	32	26	6

May use 1 piece of bread to decrease carbs and add a small salad to increase fiber.

(A "plain 'ole sandwich" can be a great meal.)

Food Source	Protein	Carbs	Fat
4 oz. tuna	30	0	0
1 tbsp. light mayo	0	2	3
Small salad (varies)	0	10	0
5 small whole wheat crackers	0	10	2
Totals	30	22	5

(Quick and easy tuna salad.)

Food Source	Protein	Carbs	Fat
3 oz. chicken breast strips	21	0	3
1 tortilla wrap (varies)	0	5	1
Lettuce, veggie condiments	0	5	0
3-4 tbsp. salsa (varies)	0	5	0
Totals	21	15	4

(Creative and delicious!)

Food Source	Protein	Carbs	Fat
Chicken breast sandwich/sub	30	35	5

Estimate well or look up in a food count book.

Ask for no mayo, no cheese.

(Everyone's on the go sometimes!)

Food Source	Protein	Carbs	Fat
Meal replacement shake	40	20	1
mixed in water			
(Not the preferable whole food lunch, but quick in a pinch.)			
Protein bar (varies)	30	30	7
(Best used as a snack so you can get fiber and whole food meals, but in an			
emergency...)			
Small salad (varies)	0	10	0
1/2 cup low-fat cottage cheese	13	4	5
Pop-top can of chicken	13	0	1
Totals	26	14	6
(Just a quick, small lunch option.)			
4 oz. baked fish	24	0	1
1 cup steamed broccoli	0	8	0
4 oz. baked potato	1	30	0
1 tsp. butter	0	0	5
Totals	25	38	6
(A great pattern for dinner.)			
1/2 oz. almonds	3	3	6
3 oz. chicken	21	0	3
1 tbsp. light mayo	0	2	3
Dash of curry (spice)	0	0	0
2 pieces whole wheat bread	6	24	0
Totals	30	29	12
(Any recipe can be used as long as the amounts of foods used are measured and			
tracked. Be creative!!)			

Snacks

Snacks are vital to your plan. They keep your blood chemistry stable (as long as your food choices are appropriate), lessen hunger, help to keep you from overeating at meals, and keep your metabolism high. Convenience, however, can compromise quality if you're not careful. To keep food quality high, snacks may be an area where you need to be more flexible with the spacing of your nutrients. For example, an apple and an eighth of a cup of almonds would make a great snack of low-glycemic carbs and quality fat, but the protein is low. Making sure your protein was adequate at your previous and your next meal would therefore be imperative. There are also a few high-quality snack bars that have a balanced amount of protein, carbs, and fat. They are especially good when you crave chocolate or a treat since there are many great flavors out there. Bars come in many sizes so stick to the right amount for your meal or snack even if you have to just eat half and save the rest for later.

After-dinner snacks can consist of a small amount of carbs or a protein shake. (Keep your eyes on those serving sizes. A bag of popcorn is three servings!) Try to keep under 150 to 200 calories per late-night snack. Weight loss will be accelerated if after-dinner snacking is eliminated or minimized, so be vigilant if you find yourself snacking too heavily at night. If you eat a protein-only snack at night, you'll decrease sleeping levels of insulin and your body will release more growth hormone at night, which increases recovery from exercise and also speeds fat loss. I'll often have a scoop of protein powder, and with some creativity it becomes like dessert. For example, after I write this paragraph, as it's 10:30 at night, I'm going straight to the kitchen, mixing a scoop of banana-flavored protein powder with a tiny amount of water in a bowl, whipping it with a fork into a cake frosting consistency, crumbling in half of a graham cracker, and it tastes just like vanilla wafer banana pudding dessert. See, creativity does pay off!

(Figure 8:3) Snacks on the Run

Food Source	Protein	Carbs	Fat
Meal replacement shake mixed in water	40	20	1
Protein bar (varies)	30	30	7
1 scoop protein powder	30	5	0
1/2 C skim milk	4	5	0
1/2 C pineapple	0	15	0
1 C strawberries	1	11	0
1 tsp. flaxseed oil	0	0	4
Totals	35	36	5
(Add ice, blend, freeze, and thaw out about one hour before eating. Tastes like frozen yogurt. Or, just blend and drink!)			
1/2 C skim milk	4	5	0
1/2 scoop protein powder	15	2	0
1 tbsp. peanut butter	5	4	8
Totals	24	11	8
(You can make an infinite variety of protein shakes!)			
"Energy/snack" bar	16	24	8
Apple	1	30	0
(Yep, just an apple can be fine. Watch out though, as a stand-alone carb source you may get hungry soon after.)			
Yogurt (per label)	10	20	3

(Figure 8:4) **Surviving Restaurants**

1) Specify how you want food prepared to avoid added butter, etc.

2) Order baked, grilled, or broiled entrees.

3) Ask for salad dressings on the side (fat-free if possible).

4) Share a meal.

5) Ask for grilled or steamed veggies instead of potato or rice if reducing carbohydrates.

6) Use red sauces instead of cream sauces.

7) Ask for cheese, croutons, bacon, egg yolks, and nuts to be left off salad.

8) Dip fork in dressing instead of pouring dressing on salad.

9) Ask for complimentary bread or chips to not be brought to the table.

10) Use a food count book to plan and estimate food intake.

11) Ask for a nutrition facts card/menu or go to the website of your favorite restaurants so you have accurate information for your log book. That way you'll never be caught off guard.

Diet Doc Cheat Sheets

As I mentioned way back in chapter two, long-term success has to be preceded at some point by you knowing enough about food counts that you can be comfortable making the right decisions in any circumstance. In other words you shouldn't be paralyzed with the question, "What should I eat?" if you find yourself outside of your normal routine. Many people falsely believe that if they have a "perfect day" planned out for them, they can follow that and be fine. A client that I've worked with for some time was having a confidence crisis recently and though she had done quite well she begged for me to create a day she could simply follow. Within two days she asked, "Can I change meal two to this…?" A day later she asked, "Since on this day I don't wake up until this time is it okay to rearrange my meals like this…?" I laughed and told her, "YES!! That's my point; you can and should change anything you want to be flexible. That's the whole idea." In contrast, I was having dinner with another client just last night who said that she felt empowered by having that flexibility and it gave her a sense of freedom that she never had dieting before and she found herself gradually becoming more creative. That, my friends, is what it's all about.

I do, however, realize that it can be easier with a starting point. I originally included sample meals to an earlier edition of my book to help readers out of the gate with some ideas. In the next edition I added a recipe section. Now, I've decided to go all out and include an actual entire day for each of the demographic categories of The Diet Doc Rx. Don't make the mistake of thinking you can follow it and eat the same thing every day, but use it for ideas to construct a good starting day for you. Exchange one food you like for another, rearrange the meal pattern to fit your schedule, and you'll be on your way to learning to stay in your ranges with the foods you enjoy and you'll gain valuable knowledge.

I used similar meals and meal patterns for the male and female charts within the same height range and often repeated them for the next level just to show how you can easily add or subtract to a meal to make it higher or lower in certain macronutrients. Every couple of height levels I completely changed the foods to show more variety. My goal was to show how effortless it is to adjust amounts but how you have the freedom to entirely change a meal.

(Figure 8:5) Personal Macronutrient Range

Men 5' - 5'4"

110 - 130 grams of protein per day
130 - 160 grams of carbohydrate per day
40 - 45 grams of fat per day

MEAL	TIME	PORTION SIZE	FOOD CONSUMED PER MEAL	Pro	Carb	Fat
1		3/1	egg whites/ whole egg	19	0	6
		2 slices	whole-grain toast	4	28	4
2			Apple or other fruit	1	24	0
3		4 oz.	chicken or turkey breast	28	0	4
			Salad (no cheese, bacon, croutons, or nuts)	0	15	0
		2 tbsp.	Italian dressing (varies)	0	3	7
4			Low-sugar yogurt	10	20	0
		1 oz.	almonds	6	6	14
5		4 oz.	chicken breast or fish	28	0	4
		2 cups	steamed vegetable such as broccoli	0	8	0
		3/4 cup	sweet potato, rice, or potato	2	36	0
6			Protein shake (varies)	20	3	2
			TOTALS FOR DAY	118	143	43

(Figure 8:6) Personal Macronutrient Range

MEAL	TIME	PORTION SIZE	FOOD CONSUMED PER MEAL	TOTAL GRAMS		
				Pro	Carb	Fat
1		1/1	egg whites/ whole egg	11	.0	6
		1 slice	whole-grain toast	2	14	2
2			Apple or other fruit	1	24	0
3		1/2 cup	low-fat cottage cheese	15	7	3
			Salad (no cheese, bacon, croutons, or nuts)	0	15	0
			Low-fat dressing	0	3	2
4			Protein shake (varies)	20	3	2
5		4 oz.	chicken breast or fish	28	0	4
		2 cups	steamed vegetable such as broccoli	0	8	0
		1/2 cup	sweet potato, rice, or potato	1	24	0
6			Rice cake	0	7	0
		1 tbsp.	peanut butter	4	4	8
			TOTALS FOR DAY	82	109	21

Women 5' - 5'4"

70 - 90 grams of protein per day
90 - 120 grams of carbohydrate per day
25 - 30 grams of fat per day

(Figure 8:7) Personal Macronutrient Range

Men 5'4" - 5'8"

120 - 140 grams of protein per day
140 - 170 grams of carbohydrate per day
45 - 50 grams of fat per day

MEAL	TIME	PORTION SIZE	FOOD CONSUMED PER MEAL	TOTAL GRAMS		
				Pro	Carb	Fat
1		1/2 cup	cup oats	5	27	3
		8 oz.	skim milk	8	4	2
2			Protein shake (varies)	20	3	2
3		4 oz.	chicken or turkey breast	28	0	4
		1 slice	cheese	7	0	7
		2 slices	whole-grain bread	4	28	4
			lettuce/tomato	0	3	0
4			Energy bar (varies)	15	25	6
5		6 oz.	chicken breast or fish	42	0	6
			Salad (no cheese, bacon, croutons, or nuts)	0	15	0
		2 tbsp.	Italian dressing (varies)	0	3	7
		1/2 cup	sweet potato, rice, or potato	1	24	0
6		3 cups	light pop corn	2	20	3
			TOTALS FOR DAY	132	152	44

91

(Figure 8:8) **Personal Macronutrient Range**

Women 5'4" - 5'8"

80 - 100 grams of protein per day
100 - 130 grams of carbohydrate per day
30 - 35 grams of fat per day

MEAL	TIME	PORTION SIZE	FOOD CONSUMED PER MEAL	TOTAL GRAMS		
				Pro	Carb	Fat
1		1/2 cup	cup oats	5	21	3
		8 oz.	skim milk	8	4	2
2			Protein shake (varies)	20	3	2
3		3 oz.	chicken breast	21	0	3
			Tortilla wrap (varies)	0	5	1
			Lettuce/tomato	0	3	0
		1 cup	strawberries	1	11	1
4			Low-sugar yogurt	10	20	0
		1/2 oz.	almonds	3	3	7
5		3 oz.	chicken breast or fish	21	0	3
			Salad (no cheese, bacon, croutons, or nuts)	0	15	0
		2 tbso.	Italian dressing (varies)	0	3	7
6		3 cups	light pop corn	2	20	3
			TOTALS FOR DAY	91	114	33

(Figure 8:9) Personal Macronutrient Range

Men 5'9" - 6'

130 - 150 grams of protein per day
150 - 180 grams of carbohydrate per day
50 - 55 grams of fat per day

MEAL	TIME	PORTION SIZE	FOOD CONSUMED PER MEAL	TOTAL GRAMS		
				Pro	Carb	Fat
1		1 scoop	protein powder (varies)	20	3	2
		1/2 tbsp.	flaxseed oil	0	0	6
			Banana	1	29	0
2			Energy bar (varies)	15	25	6
3		3 oz.	chicken breast sub	27	45	6
4			Apple	1	24	0
		1 tbsp.	peanut butter	4	4	8
5		6 oz.	chicken breast or fish	42	0	6
		2 cups	steamed vegetable medley	0	8	0
		1	dinner roll	1	22	4
6		1 scoop	protein powder (varies)	20	3	2
		1 tbsp.	peanut butter	4	4	8
			TOTALS FOR DAY	135	167	49

(Figure 8:10) **Personal Macronutrient Range**

Women 5'9" - 6'

90 - 110 grams of protein per day
110 - 140 grams of carbohydrate per day
35 - 40 grams of fat per day

MEAL	TIME	PORTION SIZE	FOOD CONSUMED PER MEAL	TOTAL GRAMS		
				Pro	Carb	Fat
1		1 scoop	protein powder (varies)	20	3	2
		1/2 tbsp.	flaxseed oil	0	0	6
		1/2 cup	blueberries	0	9	0
2			Energy bar (varies)	15	25	6
3		3 oz.	chicken breast wrap	15	25	5
4			Apple	1	24	0
5		3 oz.	chicken breast or fish	21	0	3
		2 cups	steamed vegetable medley	0	8	0
		1	dinner roll	1	22	4
6		1 scoop	protein powder (varies)	20	3	2
		1 tbsp.	peanut butter	4	4	8
			TOTALS FOR DAY	106	123	37

(Figure 8:11) Personal Macronutrient Range

Men 6' - 6'4"

140 - 160 grams of protein per day
160 - 190 grams of carbohydrate per day
55 - 60 grams of fat per day

MEAL	TIME	PORTION SIZE	FOOD CONSUMED PER MEAL	TOTAL GRAMS		
				Pro	Carb	Fat
1		1 cup	high-fiber cereal (varies)	3	35	1
		1 cup	skim milk	8	4	2
		1 scoop	protein powder (varies)	20	3	2
2			Granola bar (varies)	4	22	3
3		3 oz.	chicken breast sub	27	45	6
		1 slice	cheese	7	0	1
		1 oz.	baked chips	1	22	3
4			Protein bar (varies)	30	30	10
5		8 oz.	lean beef	48	0	16
			salad (no cheese, bacon, croutons, or nuts)	0	15	0
		2 tbsp.	Italian dressing (varies)	0	3	1
6						
			TOTALS FOR DAY	148	179	51

(Figure 8:12) Personal Macronutrient Range

MEAL	TIME	PORTION SIZE	FOOD CONSUMED PER MEAL	TOTAL GRAMS		
				Pro	Carb	Fat
1		3/4 cup	high-fiber cereal (varies)	2	26	1
		1 cup	skim milk	8	4	2
		1 scoop	protein powder (varies)	20	3	2
2			Orange	1	21	0
3		3 oz.	chicken breast sub	21	45	6
		1 slice	cheese	7	0	1
4			Granola bar (varies)	4	22	3
5		6 oz.	lean beef	36	0	12
			Salad (no cheese, bacon, croutons, or nuts)	0	15	0
		2 tbsp.	Italian dressing (varies)	0	3	1
6						
			TOTALS FOR DAY	105	139	40

Women 6' - 6'4"

100 - 120 grams of protein per day
120 - 150 grams of carbohydrate per day
40 - 45 grams of fat per day

RECIPES

DINNERS

Southwest Chicken

4 boneless skinless chicken breast halves (1 pound)

16 ounces picante sauce

2 tablespoons brown sugar

1 tablespoon mustard

Place chicken in a greased shallow 2-qt. baking dish. In a small bowl, combine the picante sauce, brown sugar, and mustard; pour over chicken. Bake, uncovered, at 400 degrees for 30-35 minutes. Serve over rice if desired.

Yield: 4 servings

Nutritional Analysis: One serving (calculated without rice) equals 224 calories, 4 g fat, 19 g carbohydrate, 28 g protein

Diabetic Exchanges: 3 lean meat, ½ starch

Light Turkey Salad Tortillas

12 ounces cooked turkey, shredded or cubed

1 cup (4 ounces) fat-free shredded cheddar cheese

¾ cup finely chopped celery

½ cup finely chopped onion

1 can (2 ¼ ounces) sliced olives, drained

½ cup light mayonnaise

¼ cup picante sauce

6 low-carb flour tortillas (7 inches)

In a bowl, combine the first 7 ingredients, mix well. Evenly divide filling on center on each tortilla. Fold sides and ends over filling, then roll up. Place in a shallow, microwave-safe dish. Cover and microwave on high for 2-3 minutes or until cheese is melted and filling is hot.

Yield: 6 servings

Nutritional Analysis: One serving equals 151 calories, 3 g fat, 16 g carbohydrate, 15 g protein

Diabetic Exchanges: ½ starch, 1 ½ meat, 1 vegetable

Lean Swedish Meatballs

2 egg whites, lightly beaten

¼ cup ketchup

¾ cup dry bread crumbs

2 tablespoons dried parsley flakes

2 tablespoons Worcestershire sauce

1 teaspoon onion powder

1 teaspoon garlic powder

1 teaspoon pepper

½ teaspoon salt

½ teaspoon chili powder

3 pounds ground turkey breast

ADDITIONAL INGREDIENTS:

2 envelopes brown gravy mix

½ cup fat-free sour cream

In a bowl, combine the first 10 ingredients. Crumble meat over mixture and mix well. Shape into 1-in. balls (about 6 dozen). Place in a single layer in ungreased 15-in. x 10-in. x 1-in. baking pans. Bake at 400 degrees for 20 minutes or until no longer pink, turning often. Remove from the oven; stir in sour cream. Cool.

Yield: 75 meatballs per batch, 15 servings

Nutritional Analysis: Five Swedish meatballs equal 223 calories, 7 g fat, 8 g carbohydrate, 32 g protein

Diabetic Exchanges: 4 lean meat, ½ starch

Blueberry Chicken

4 boneless skinless chicken breast halves (1 pound)

1 tablespoon canola oil

¼ cup apricot preserves *or* fruit spread

3 tablespoons Dijon mustard

¼ cup white wine vinegar *or* cider vinegar

1 cup fresh *or* frozen blueberries

In a large skillet over medium heat, cook chicken in oil for about 5 minutes on each side or until lightly browned. Combine preserves and mustard; spoon over chicken. Reduce heat to low; cover and simmer for 20 minutes or until chicken juices run clear.

With a slotted spoon, remove chicken and keep warm. Add vinegar to skillet; bring to a boil. Reduce heat, simmer uncovered for 3 minutes or until sauce is reduced by one-third, stirring occasionally. Stir in blueberries. Serve rice if desired.

Yield: 4 servings

Nutritional Analysis: One serving (prepared with 100% apricot fruit spread) equals 206 calories, 6 g fat, 10 g carbohydrate, 28 g protein

Diabetic Exchanges: 3 lean meat, 1 1/2 fruit

Creamy Chicken Enchiladas

1 small onion, chopped

1 can (10 ¾ ounces) reduced-fat, reduced-sodium condensed cream of chicken soup, undiluted

1 can (10 ounces) diced tomatoes and green chilies, undrained

1 cup (8 ounces) fat-free sour cream

1 cup (4 ounces) shredded fat-free cheddar cheese

1 cup (4 ounces) shredded reduced-fat mozzarella cheese

6 low-carb flour tortillas

3 cooked chicken breasts (cubed)

In a skillet or saucepan coated with nonstick cooking spray, sauté onion until tender. Remove from heat. Add soup, tomatoes, sour cream, ¾ cup cheddar cheese, and ¾ cup mozzarella cheese; mix well. Divide evenly on each tortilla, top with ½ of a cubed chicken breast. Roll up tightly.

Place seam side down in a 13-in. x 9-in. x 2-in. baking dish coated with nonstick cooking spray. Top with remaining soup mixture; sprinkle with remaining cheeses. Bake, uncovered, at 350 degrees for 20-25 minutes or until heated through.

Yield: 6 servings

Nutritional Analysis: One serving equals 226 calories, 6 g fat, 21 g carbohydrate, 22 g protein

Diabetic Exchanges: 2 lean meat, 1 ½ starch, 1 vegetable

Dill Salmon

1 salmon fillet (1 pound)

1 ½ teaspoons dill weed

½ cup fat-free plain yogurt

½ teaspoon brown sugar

½ teaspoon salt-free seasoning blend

Place the salmon in a 13-in. x 9-in. x 2-in. baking dish coated with nonstick cooking spray and sprinkle with ½ teaspoon dill. Cover and bake at 375 degrees for 20-25 minutes or until the fish flakes easily with a fork. In a small saucepan, combine the yogurt, sugar, seasoning blend, and remaining dill. Cook and stir over low heat until heated through.

Yield: 4 servings

Nutritional Analysis: One serving equals 227 calories, 12 g fat, 3 g carbohydrate, 24 g protein

Diabetic Exchanges: 2 ½ lean meat, 2 fat.

Lean and Meaty Spaghetti Sauce

1 ½ pounds ground turkey breast

½ pound bulk Italian sausage

1 medium green pepper, chopped

1 medium onion, chopped

8 garlic cloves, minced

3 cans (14 1/2 ounces *each*) diced tomatoes, drained

2 cans (15 ounces *each*) tomato sauce

2 cans (6 ounces *each*) tomato paste

¼ cup sugar

2 tablespoons Italian seasoning

1 tablespoon dried basil

1 teaspoon salt

½ teaspoon pepper

Hot cooked spaghetti

In a large skillet over medium heat, cook turkey and sausage until no longer pink; drain. Transfer to a 5-qt. slower cooker. Stir in green pepper, onion, garlic, tomatoes, tomato sauce, paste, sugar, and seasonings; mix well. Cover and cook on low for 8 hours or until bubbly. Serve over spaghetti.

Yield: 12 servings

Nutritional Analysis: One serving (calculated without spaghetti – add macronutrient values for amount of spaghetti served) equals 180 calories, 4 g fat, 12 g carbohydrate, 24 g protein

Diabetic Exchanges: 1 starch, 2 meat, 1 vegetable

Italian Orange Roughy Fillets

1 pound orange roughy fillets

½ cup tomato juice

1 tablespoon white vinegar

1 envelope Italian salad dressing mix

¼ cup chopped green onions

¼ cup chopped green pepper

Place fish fillets in a shallow 2-qt glass baking dish, positioning the thickest portion of fish toward the outside edges. Combine tomato juice, vinegar, and salad dressing mix; pour over fish. Cover and refrigerate for 30 minutes.

Sprinkle with onions and green pepper. Cover and bake at 400 for 15 minutes or until fish flakes easily with a fork. Let stand, covered, for 2 minutes.

Yield: 4 servings

Nutritional Analysis: One serving equals 122 calories, 2 g fat, 5 g carbohydrate, 21 g protein

Diabetic Exchanges: 2 very lean meat

Oriental Sesame Chicken

1 pound boneless skinless chicken breasts, cubed

1 tablespoon canola oil

¼ cup light soy sauce

¼ cup sesame seeds

1 large onion, sliced

2 jars (4 1/2 ounces *each*) sliced mushrooms, drained, *or* 2 cups sliced fresh mushrooms

In a large skillet, cook chicken in oil until no longer pink. Stir in the soy sauce and sesame seeds. Cook and stir over medium heat for 5 minutes. Remove chicken with a slotted spoon; set aside and keep warm. In the same skillet, sauté onion and mushrooms until onion is tender. Return chicken to pan; heat through.

Yield: 4 servings

Nutritional Analysis: One serving equals 212 calories, 8 g fat, 6 g carbohydrate, 29 g protein

Diabetic Exchange: 4 very lean meat, 1 fat, 1 vegetable

Light Spinach Quiche

3 ounces fat-free cream cheese

1 cup skim milk

8 egg whites

¼ teaspoon pepper

3 cups (12 ounces) shredded fat-free cheddar cheese

1 package (10 ounces) frozen chopped spinach, thawed and squeezed dry

1 cup frozen chopped broccoli, thawed and well-drained

1 small onion, finely chopped

5 fresh mushrooms, sliced

In a small mixing bowl, beat cream cheese. Add milk, egg whites, and pepper; beat until smooth. Stir in remaining ingredients. Transfer to a 10-in quiche pan coated with nonstick cooking spray. Bake at 350 degrees for 45-50 minutes or until a knife inserted near the center comes out clean.

Yield: 8 servings

Nutritional Analysis: One serving equals 122 calories, 2 g fat, 8 g carbohydrate, 18 g protein

Diabetic Exchanges: 1 starch, 1 meat

Italian Chicken Cutlets

6 boneless skinless chicken breast halves (1 ½ pounds)

1 cup dry bread crumbs

½ cup nonfat Parmesan cheese topping

2 tablespoons wheat germ

1 teaspoon dried basil

½ teaspoon garlic powder

1 cup plain fat-free yogurt

Refrigerated butter-flavored spray

Flatten chicken to ½-in. thickness. In a shallow dish, combine the bread crumbs, Parmesan topping, wheat germ, basil, and garlic powder. Place the yogurt in another shallow dish. Dip chicken in yogurt, then coat with the crumb mixture. Place in a 15-in. x 10-in. x 1-in. baking pan coated with nonstick cooking spray. Spritz chicken with butter-flavored spray. Bake, uncovered, at 350 degrees for 20-25 minutes or until the juices run clear.

Yield: 6 servings

Nutritional Analysis: One serving equals 270 calories, 5 g fat, 15 g carbohydrate, 32 g protein

Diabetic Exchanges: 3 lean meat, 1 starch

Chicken Veggie Stew

2 pounds boneless skinless chicken breasts, cubed

1 can (14 ½ ounces) Italian diced tomatoes, undrained

2 medium potatoes, peeled and cut into ½ inch cubes

6 medium carrots, chopped

4 celery stalks, chopped

1 large onion, chopped

1 medium green pepper, chopped

2 cans (4 ounces *each*) mushrooms, drained

2 low-sodium chicken bouillon cubes

1 teaspoon chili powder

¼ teaspoon pepper

1 tablespoon cornstarch

2 cups water

In a slow cooker, combine the first 11 ingredients. In a small bowl, combine cornstarch and water until smooth. Stir into chicken mixture. Cover and cook on low for 8-10 hours or until vegetables are tender.

Yield: 8 servings

Nutritional Analysis: One serving equals 220 calories, 4 g fat, 16 g carbohydrate, 30 g protein

Diabetic Exchanges: 2 vegetable, 3 lean meat, ½ starch

Spicy White Chili

2 pounds boneless skinless chicken breasts, cubed

1 small onion, chopped

2 cups low-sodium chicken broth

1 can (4 ounces) chopped green chilies

½ teaspoon garlic powder

½ teaspoon dried oregano

½ teaspoon minced fresh cilantro *or* parsley

¼ teaspoon cayenne pepper

1 can (15 ounces) white kidney or cannelini beans, rinsed and drained

In a saucepan coated with nonstick cooking spray, sauté chicken and onion until juices run clear; drain if desired. Stir in broth, chilies, garlic powder, oregano, cilantro, and cayenne. Bring to a boil. Reduce heat; simmer, uncovered, for 30 minutes. Stir in beans; cook 10 minutes longer.

Yield: 8 servings

Nutritional Analysis: One serving equals 220 calories, 4 g fat, 14 g carbohydrate, 32 g protein

Diabetic Exchanges: 3 ½ lean meat, 1 starch, 1 vegetable

Zesty Cod

1 ½ cups water

1 tablespoon lemon juice

2 pounds cod fillets

¼ tsp pepper

1 small onion, finely chopped

2 large tomatoes, sliced

½ cup chopped green pepper

½ cup seasoned bread crumbs

¼ cup grated, reduced-fat Parmesan cheese

½ teaspoon dried basil

1 tablespoon olive oil

In a bowl, combine the water and lemon juice. Add fish; let sit for 5 minutes. Drain and place in an 11-in. x 7-in. x 2-in. baking dish coated with nonstick cooking spray. Sprinkle with pepper. Layer with onion, tomatoes, and green pepper. Combine the remaining ingredients, sprinkle over top. Bake, uncovered, at 375 degrees for 20-30 minutes or until fish flakes easily with a fork.

Yield: 8 servings

Nutritional Analysis: One serving equals 188 calories, 4 g fat, 10 g carbohydrate, 28 g protein

Diabetic Exchanges: 3 lean meat, 1 starch

Creamed Mushroom Turkey

1 boneless turkey breast (3 pounds), halved

1 tablespoon canola oil-based butter, melted

2 tablespoons dried parsley flakes

½ teaspoon dried tarragon

½ teaspoon salt

¼ teaspoon pepper

1 jar (4 ½ ounces) sliced mushrooms, drained *or* 1 cup sliced fresh mushrooms

½ cup chicken broth

2 tablespoons cornstarch

¼ cup cold water

Place the turkey in a slow cooker. Brush with butter. Sprinkle with parsley, tarragon, salt, and pepper. Top with mushrooms. Pour broth over all. Cover and cook on low for 7-8 hours. Remove turkey and keep warm. Skim fat from cooking juices. In a saucepan, combine cornstarch and water until smooth. Gradually add cooking juices. Bring to a boil; cook and stir for 2 minutes or until thickened. Serve over the turkey.

Yield: 12 servings

Nutritional Analysis: One serving equals 191 calories, 7 g fat, 4 g carbohydrate, 28 g protein

Diabetic Exchanges: 3 lean meat, ½ vegetable

Curry Chicken Breasts

4 boneless skinless chicken breast halves (4 ounces each)

1 tablespoon canola oil

¼ cup Worcestershire sauce

2 tablespoons chili sauce

2 teaspoons curry powder

1 teaspoon garlic powder

¼ teaspoon hot pepper sauce

¼ cup chopped onion

In a large skillet, brown chicken on both sides in oil. In a bowl, combine the Worcestershire sauce, chili sauce, curry powder, garlic powder, and hot pepper sauce. Pour over chicken. Add onion. Reduce heat; cover and simmer for 9-11 minutes.

Yield: 4 servings

Nutritional Analysis: One serving equals 186 calories, 6 g fat, 4 g carbohydrate, 28 g protein

Diabetic Exchanges: 3 lean meat, 1 vegetable

Parmesan Chicken

½ cup dry bread crumbs

½ cup grated reduced-fat Parmesan cheese

2 tablespoons minced fresh parsley

1 garlic clove, minced

¼ teaspoon pepper

4 egg whites

8 boneless skinless chicken breast halves (2 pounds)

½ cup sliced almonds

Butter-flavored cooking spray

In a shallow bowl, combine the first 5 ingredients. In another shallow bowl, beat the egg whites. Dip chicken in egg whites, then coat with crumb mixture. Place in a 13-in. x 9-in. x 2-in. baking dish coated with nonstick cooking spray. Sprinkle almonds over chicken. Spritz lightly with butter-flavored spray. Bake, uncovered, at 350 degrees for 30 minutes.

Yield: 8 servings

Nutritional Analysis: One serving equals 216 calories, 8 g fat, 6 g carbohydrate, 30 g protein

Diabetic Exchanges: 3 lean meat, ½ starch

Mini Turkey Loaves

4 egg whites

½ cup fat-free plain yogurt

1 can (6 ounces) tomato paste

2 tablespoons Worcestershire sauce

½ cup quick-cooking oats

1 small onion, chopped

2 tablespoons dried parsley flakes

1 teaspoon salt

½ teaspoon garlic powder

½ teaspoon pepper

2 pounds ground turkey breast

½ cup low-carb ketchup

In a large bowl, combine the first 10 ingredients. Crumble turkey over mixture and mix well. Shape into eight loaves. Place on a rack coated with nonstick cooking spray in a shallow baking pan. Bake, uncovered, at 350 degrees for 30 minutes. Spoon ketchup over the loaves. Bake 15 minutes longer.

Yield: 8 servings

Nutritional Analysis: One serving equals 172 calories, 4 g fat, 2 g carbohydrates, 30 g protein

Diabetic Exchanges: 3 lean meat, 1 starch, ½ fat

Sweet and Spicy Chicken

1 pound boneless skinless chicken breasts, cut into ½ inch cubes

3 tablespoons taco seasoning

1 tablespoon canola oil

1 jar (11 ounces) chunky salsa

½ cup sugar-free peach preserves

Coat chicken with taco seasoning. In a skillet, brown chicken in oil. Combine salsa and preserves; stir into skillet. Bring to a boil. Reduce heat; cover and simmer for 2-3 minutes. Serve over rice if desired.

Yield: 4 servings

Nutritional Analysis: One serving equals 197 calories, 5 g fat, 10 g carbohydrate, 28 g protein

Diabetic Exchanges: 3 lean meat, 1 fruit, ½ fat

Lemon Baked Salmon

1 salmon fillet (2 pounds)

2 tablespoons canola oil-based butter

¼ cup white wine

2 tablespoons lemon juice

½ teaspoon pepper

½ teaspoon dried tarragon

Sliced lemon

Pat salmon dry. Place in a greased 13-in. x 9-in. x 2-in. baking dish. Brush with butter. Combine remaining ingredients; pour over salmon. Top salmon with lemon slices. Bake, uncovered, at 425 degrees for 20-25 minutes or until fish flakes easily with a fork.

Yield: 8 servings

Nutritional Analysis: One (4-ounce) serving equals 192 calories, 8 g fat, 2 g carbohydrate, 28 g protein

Diabetic Exchanges: 4 lean meat, 1 fat

Orange Roughy Primavera

1 tablespoon canola oil-based butter

4 orange roughy fillets (4 ounces each), thawed

2 tablespoons lemon juice

Pinch pepper

1 garlic clove, minced

1 tablespoon olive oil

1 cup broccoli florets

1 cup cauliflowerets

1 cup julienned carrots

1 cup sliced fresh mushrooms

½ cup sliced celery

¼ teaspoon dried basil

¼ teaspoon salt

¼ cup reduced-fat, grated Parmesan cheese

Place butter in a 13-in. x 9-in. x 2-in. baking dish; add fish and turn to coat. Sprinkle with lemon juice and pepper. Bake, uncovered, at 450 degrees for 5 minutes. Meanwhile, in a large skillet over medium heat, sauté garlic in oil. Add the next 7 ingredients, stir-fry until vegetables are crisp-tender, about 2-3 minutes. Spoon over the fish; sprinkle with cheese. Bake, uncovered, at 450 degrees for 3-5 minutes or until fish flakes easily with a fork.

Yield: 4 servings

Nutritional Analysis: One serving equals 215 calories, 7 g fat, 10 g carbohydrate, 28 g protein

Diabetic Exchanges: 3 very lean meat, 1 ½ vegetable, 1 fat

Spicy Haddock

2 pounds haddock fillets, thawed

1 can (4 ounces) chopped green chilies

1 tablespoon canola oil

1 tablespoon soy sauce

2 tablespoons Worcestershire sauce

1 teaspoon paprika

½ teaspoon garlic powder

½ teaspoon chili powder

Dash hot pepper sauce

Place fillets in a 13-in. x 9-in. x 2-in. baking dish that has been coated with nonstick cooking spray. Combine remaining ingredients; spoon over fish. Bake, uncovered, at 350 degrees for 20-25 minutes or until fish flakes easily with a fork.

Yield: 8 servings

Nutritional Analysis: One (4-ounce) serving equals 155 calories, 5 g fat, 2 g carbohydrate, 28 g protein

Diabetic Exchanges: 3 very lean meat, ½ vegetable

Lemon Fish

1 pound whitefish *or* sole fillets

¼ cup lemon juice

1 teaspoon olive oil

2 teaspoons salt-free lemon-pepper seasoning

1 small onion, thinly sliced

1 teaspoon dried parsley flakes

Cut fish into serving-size pieces. Place in an ungreased 11-in. x 7-in. x 2-in. baking dish. Drizzle with lemon juice and oil; sprinkle with lemon pepper.

Arrange onion over fish; sprinkle with parsley. Cover and let stand for 5 minutes. Bake at 350 degrees for 20 minutes or until fish flakes easily with a fork.

Yield: 4 servings

Nutritional Analysis: One serving equals 156 calories, 6 g fat, 2 g carbohydrate, 28 g protein

Diabetic Exchanges: 3 very lean meat

Turkey Tortilla Pie

1 small onion, finely chopped

½ teaspoon garlic powder

1 teaspoon olive oil

1 pound ground turkey breast

2 teaspoons chili powder

1 teaspoon dried oregano

½ teaspoon ground cumin

½ teaspoon cayenne pepper

1 can (15 ounces) black beans, rinsed and drained

1 jar (16 ounces) salsa

¾ cup low-sodium chicken broth

8 low-carb, fat-free flour tortillas

½ cup shredded reduced-fat Monterey Jack cheese

¼ cup light sour cream

In a skillet, sauté onion and garlic powder in oil until the onion is tender. Add turkey, chili powder, oregano, cumin, and cayenne, cook and stir over medium heat until turkey is no longer pink. Stir in beans. Remove from heat. Combine salsa and broth; spread a thin layer in a 2 ½-qt. baking dish coated with nonstick cooking spray. Cut tortillas into 1 inch strips and then into thirds; arrange half over salsa mixture. Top with half of the turkey mixture and half of the remaining salsa mixture. Repeat layers. Sprinkle with cheese. Cover and bake at 350 degrees for 25 minutes or until bubbly. Top servings with sour cream.

Yield: 8 servings

Nutritional Analysis: One (1 cup) serving equals 270 calories, 6 g fat, 32 g carbohydrate, 22 g protein

Diabetic Exchanges: 2 starch, 2 lean meat, 1 vegetable

Italian-Tomato Chicken

4 boneless skinless chicken breast halves (1 pound)

½ cup fat-free Italian salad dressing

8 tomato slices, ¼ inch thick

4 teaspoons seasoned bread crumbs

1 teaspoon minced fresh basil *or* ¼ teaspoon dried basil

1 tablespoon grated, reduced-fat Parmesan cheese

Place chicken in a shallow bowl; pour ¼ cup dressing over chicken. Cover and refrigerate for 2 hours. Transfer chicken to a shallow baking dish; discard marinade. Drizzle with remaining dressing. Cover and bake at 400 degrees for 10 minutes. Top each chicken breast with tomato slices, crumbs, basil, and cheese. Cover and bake for 10 minutes. Uncover and bake 10-15 minutes longer or until chicken juices run clear.

Yield: 4 servings

Nutritional Analysis: One serving equals 164 calories, 4 g fat, 8 g carbohydrate, 28 g protein

Diabetic Exchanges: 3 lean meat, ½ starch

Creamy Pea Salad

2 medium carrots, chopped

1 package (16 ounces) frozen peas

1 celery rib, thinly sliced

¼ cup cubed reduced-fat mozzarella cheese

2 green onions, thinly sliced

2 tablespoons buttermilk

2 tablespoons plain nonfat yogurt

1 teaspoon fat-free mayonnaise

½ teaspoon cider *or* red wine vinegar

½ teaspoon dried basil

¼ teaspoon pepper

In a saucepan, cook carrots in a small amount of boiling water for 2 minutes. Add peas; cook 5 minutes longer. Drain; rinse in cold water and drain again. Place in a bowl; add celery, cheese, and onions. Combine remaining ingredients; pour over pea mixture and toss to coat. Cover and refrigerate for at least 1 hour.

Yield: 5 servings

Nutritional Analysis: One (¾ cup) serving equals 103 calories, 3 g fat, 15 g carbohydrate, 4 g protein

Diabetic Exchanges: 1 vegetable, ½ starch

Cilantro Lime Cod

4 cod fillets (2 pounds)

¼ teaspoon pepper

1 tablespoon dried minced onion

1 garlic clove, minced

1 tablespoon olive oil

1 teaspoon ground cumin

¼ cup minced fresh cilantro *or* parsley

2 limes, thinly sliced

1 tablespoon canola oil-based butter

Place each fillet on a 15-in. x 12-in. piece of heavy-duty foil. Sprinkle with pepper. In a small saucepan, sauté onion and garlic in oil; stir in cumin. Spoon over fillets; spinkle with cilantro. Place lime slices over each; drizzle with butter. Fold foil around fish and seal tightly. Place on a baking sheet. Bake at 375 degrees for 35-40 minutes or until fish flakes easily with a fork.

Yield: 8 servings

Nutritional Analysis: One serving equals 209 calories, 6 g fat, 3 g carbohydrate, 28 g protein

Diabetic Exchanges: 2 very lean meat, ½ fat

Chicken Burritos

¼ cup olive oil

¼ cup lime juice

4 garlic cloves, minced

1 tablespoon minced fresh parsley or 1 teaspoon dried parsley flakes

1 teaspoon ground cumin

1 teaspoon dried oregano

¼ teaspoon pepper

4 boneless skinless chicken breast halves (1 pound)

6 low-carb, fat-free flour tortillas

Shredded lettuce, diced tomatoes, and other vegetable condiments of your choice

In a large resealable plastic bag or shallow glass container, combine the first 7 ingredients. Add chicken and turn to coat. Seal or cover and refrigerate 8 hours or overnight, turning occasionally. Drain and discard marinade. Grill chicken, uncovered, over medium heat for 5-7 minutes on each side or until juices run clear. Cut into thin strips; serve in tortillas or taco shells with desired vegetable condiments.

Yield: 6 servings

Nutritional Analysis: One serving equals 201 calories, 5 g fat, 15 g carbohydrate, 24 g protein

Diabetic Exchanges: 3 lean meat, 1 starch, ½ fat

Lemon Chicken

½ cup water

¼ cup lemon juice

2 tablespoons dried minced onion

1 tablespoon dried parsley flakes

1 tablespoon Worcestershire sauce

1 garlic clove, minced

1 teaspoon dill seed

½ teaspoon curry powder

½ teaspoon pepper

8 boneless skinless chicken breast halves (2 pounds), cut up

In a large resealable bag or shallow glass container, combine the first 9 ingredients. Add chicken and turn to coat. Seal or cover and refrigerate for 4-6 hours. Drain and discard marinade. Grill chicken, covered, over low heat for 50-60 minutes or until juices run clear, turning several times.

Yield: 8 servings

Nutritional Analysis: One serving equals 156 calories, 4 g fat, 2 g carbohydrates, 28 g protein

Diabetic Exchanges: 3 lean meat

Cajun Salmon Steaks

2 salmon steaks (6 ounces, 1 inch thick)

½ teaspoon Worcestershire sauce

½ teaspoon lemon juice

½ teaspoon Cajun *or* Creole seasoning

½ cup diced green pepper

½ cup diced red pepper

Place the salmon in an ungreased 8-in. square microwave-safe dish. Rub with Worcestershire sauce and lemon juice; sprinkle with Cajun seasoning. Sprinkle peppers on top. Cover and microwave on high for 5-6 minutes, turning once, or until fish flakes easily with a fork. Let stand, covered, for 1 minute.

Yield: 2 servings

Nutritional Analysis: One serving equals 268 calories, 12 g fat, 4 g carbohydrate, 36 g protein

Diabetic Exchanges: 3 lean meat, 1 vegetable, 1 fat

Garlic Chicken

½ cup dry bread crumbs

¼ cup reduced-fat grated Parmesan cheese

2 tablespoons minced fresh parsley

¼ teaspoon pepper

¼ cup skim milk

6 boneless skinless chicken breast halves (1 ½ pounds)

¼ cup canola oil-based butter

2 garlic cloves, minced

2 tablespoons lemon juice

Pinch paprika

In a large resealable plastic bag, combine the first 5 ingredients. Place milk in a shallow bowl. Dip chicken in milk, then shake in the crumb mixture. Place in a greased 13-in. x 9-in. x 2-in. baking dish. Combine the butter, garlic, and lemon juice; drizzle over the chicken. Sprinkle with paprika. Bake, uncovered, at 350 degrees for 25-30 minutes.

Yield: 6 servings

Nutritional Analysis: One serving equals 172 calories, 6 g fat, 4 g carbohydrate, 30 g protein

Diabetic Exchanges: 3 lean meat, 1 fat, ½ starch

Chili Chicken Breasts

1 teaspoon chili powder

½ teaspoon ground cumin

¼ teaspoon garlic powder

¼ teaspoon cayenne pepper

4 boneless skinless chicken breast halves (1 pound)

1 teaspoon canola oil

¼ cup chopped green onions

1 jalapeno pepper, seeded and finely chopped

1 garlic clove, minced

1 can (14 1/2 ounces) diced tomatoes, undrained

1 teaspoon cornstarch

2 teaspoons water

Combine the first 4 ingredients, rub over chicken. In a nonstick skillet, brown chicken in oil on both sides. Add onions, jalapeno, and garlic; sauté for 1 minute. Add tomatoes; bring to a boil. Reduce heat; cover and simmer for 15-20 minutes. Remove chicken and keep warm. In a small bowl, combine cornstarch and water until smooth; stir in tomato mixture. Bring to a boil; cook and stir for 1 minute or until slightly thickened. Serve over chicken.

Yield: 4 servings

Nutritional Analysis: One serving equals 164 calories, 4 g fat, 4 g carbohydrate, 28 g protein

Diabetic Exchanges: 3 lean meat, 1 vegetable

Broccoli-Cabbage Slaw

2 cups shredded cabbage

2 cups broccoli florets

1 cup cauliflowerets

1 medium red onion, thinly sliced

¼ cup reduced-fat mayonnaise

¼ cup fat-free plain yogurt

¼ cup reduced-fat sour cream

¼ cup reduced-fat shredded Parmesan cheese

In a salad bowl, combine the cabbage, broccoli, cauliflower, and onion. In a small bowl, combine the remaining ingredients. Pour over vegetables and toss to coat. Cover and refrigerate until serving.

Yield: 6 servings

Nutritional Analysis: One (¾ cup) serving equals 116 calories, 6 g fat, 15 g carbohydrate, 5 g protein

Diabetic Exchanges: 1 vegetable, 1 fat, ½ starch

Herbed Lime Chicken

1 bottle (16 ounces) fat-free Italian salad dressing

½ cup lime juice

1 lime, halved and sliced

3 garlic cloves, minced

1 teaspoon dried thyme

8 boneless skinless chicken breast halves (2 pounds)

In a bowl, combine the first 5 ingredients. Remove ½ cup for basting; cover and refrigerate. Pour remaining marinade into a large resealable plastic bag; add chicken. Seal bag and turn to coat; refrigerate for 8-10 hours. Drain and discard marinade. Grill chicken, uncovered, over medium heat for 5 minutes. Turn chicken; baste with the reserved marinade. Grill 5-7 minutes longer, basting occasionally.

Yield: 8 servings

Nutritional Analysis: One serving equals 172 calories, 4 g fat, 6 g carbohydrate, 28 g protein

Diabetic Exchanges: 3 lean meat

Stuffed Sole

2 tablespoons canola oil-based butter

2 tablespoons lemon juice

½ teaspoon salt

¼ teaspoon pepper

1 package (10 ounces) frozen chopped broccoli, thawed and drained

1 cup cooked rice

1 cup (4 ounces) shredded reduced-fat cheddar cheese

8 sole *or* whitefish fillets (4 ounces each)

Paprika

In a small bowl, combine the butter, lemon juice, salt, and pepper. In another bowl, combine the broccoli, rice, cheese, and half of the butter mixture. Spoon ½ cup onto each fillet. Roll up and place seam side down in a baking dish coated with nonstick cooking spray. Pour remaining butter mixture over roll-ups.

Bake, uncovered, at 350 degrees for 25 minutes or until fish flakes easily with a fork. Baste with pan drippings; sprinkle with paprika.

Yield: 8 servings

Nutritional Analysis: One serving equals 231 calories, 7 g fat, 12 g carbohydrate, 30 g protein

Diabetic Exchanges: 3 lean meat, 1 vegetable, ½ starch

Mushroom Spinach Tart

2 tablespoons seasoned bread crumbs

½ pound fresh mushrooms, sliced

½ cup chopped onion

1 tablespoon olive oil

1 package (10 ounces) frozen chopped spinach, thawed and squeezed dry

1 cup skim milk

1 cup egg substitute

¼ teaspoon salt

¼ teaspoon pepper

1 cup shredded reduced-fat Mexican cheese

½ cup grated reduced-fat Parmesan cheese

Coat a 9-in. pie plate with nonstick cooking spray. Sprinkle bottom and sides with bread crumbs; shake out the excess. Set plate aside. In a nonstick skillet, sauté mushrooms and onion in oil for 12-14 minutes or until all of the liquid has evaporated. Remove from the heat; stir in spinach.

In a bowl, combine the milk, egg substitute, salt, and pepper. Stir in the spinach mixture, 1 cup Mexican cheese blend and Parmesan cheese. Pour into prepared pie plate. Bake at 350 degrees for 35-40 minutes or until a knife inserted near the center comes out clean. Sprinkle remaining cheese around edge of tart. Let stand for 5 minutes before slicing.

Yield: 8 servings

Nutritional Analysis: One piece equals 176 calories, 8 g fat, 10 g carbohydrate, 16 g protein

Diabetic Exchanges: 2 lean meat, 1 vegetable, 1 fat, ½ starch

LUNCHES

Garden Tuna Sandwiches

2 cans (6 ounces) water-packed tuna, drained

½ cup chopped peeled cucumber

½ shredded carrot

¼ cup finely chopped green onions

½ cup fat-free mayonnaise

¼ cup Dijon mustard

1 tablespoon fat-free sour cream

1 teaspoon lemon juice

¼ teaspoon pepper

8 slices whole wheat bread

4 lettuce leaves

In a bowl, combine the tuna, cucumber, carrot, onions, mayonnaise, mustard, sour cream, lemon juice, and pepper. Spread on four slices of bread; top with lettuce and remaining bread.

Yield: 4 servings

Nutritional Analysis: One sandwich equals 236 calories, 4 g fat, 32 g carbohydrate, 18 g protein

Diabetic Exchanges: 2 starch, 1 ½ lean meat, 1 vegetable

Mushroom Turkey Burger

2 pounds ground turkey breast

1 can (4 ounces) mushroom stems and pieces, drained

¼ cup egg substitute

½ cup chopped onion

¼ cup ketchup

1 teaspoon Italian seasoning

¼ teaspoon pepper

¼ teaspoon Worcestershire sauce

In a bowl, combine all ingredients. Divide into 8 patties and grill, covered, over medium heat until meat is no longer pink, turning once.

Yield: 8 servings

Nutritional Analysis: One serving equals 186 calories, 6 g fat, 4 g carbohydrate, 29 g protein

Diabetic Exchanges: 3 lean meat, 1 vegetable

Chicken Cheddar Wraps

½ cup (4 ounces) fat-free sour cream

¾ cup chunky salsa

2 tablespoons light mayonnaise

4 boneless skinless chicken breast halves (1 pound)

1 cup (4 ounces) fat-free shredded cheddar cheese

½ cup thinly sliced fresh mushrooms

2 cups shredded lettuce

6 low-carb, fat-free flour tortillas

Tomato wedges

In a bowl, combine the sour cream, salsa, and mayonnaise. Stir in chicken, cheese, and mushrooms. Divide lettuce between tortillas. Place about ½ cup chicken mixture on each tortilla. Fold sides over the fillings. Garnish with tomato.

Yield: 6 wraps

Nutritional Analysis: One wrap equals 167 calories, 3 g fat, 17 g carbohydrate, 18 g protein

Diabetic Exchanges: 1 starch, 2 lean meat, 1 vegetable

Vegetarian Burritos

10 egg whites (or equivalent egg substitute)

¼ teaspoon pepper

1 cup salsa

¼ cup chopped onion

1 cup (4 ounces) fat-free shredded cheddar cheese

8 low-carb, fat-free flour tortillas

In a bowl, beat the eggs and pepper. Pour into a skillet that has been coated with nonstick cooking spray. Cook and stir over medium heat until eggs are partially set. Add salsa and onion, cook, and stir until eggs are completely set. Sprinkle with cheese. Spoon about ½ cup down the center of each tortilla; fold ends and sides over filling. Serve immediately.

Yield: 8 servings

Nutritional Analysis: One serving equals 146 calories, 2 g fat, 20 g carbohydrate, 12 g protein

Diabetic Exchanges: 1 starch, 1 vegetable, 1 lean meat

Italian Mushroom Salad

2 pounds fresh mushrooms, quartered

3 medium tomatoes, cut into wedges

1 cup fat-free Italian salad dressing

1 teaspoon dried parsley flakes

½ teaspoon garlic powder

¼ cup chopped onion

½ teaspoon dried basil

3 cups fresh spinach leaves

4 turkey bacon strips, cooked and chopped

Place mushrooms and tomatoes in a large shallow dish. Combine the next 5 ingredients; drizzle over mushrooms and tomatoes. Cover and refrigerate overnight, stirring once. Line a serving platter or bowl with spinach. Using a slotted spoon, arrange vegetables over spinach. Sprinkle with turkey bacon.

Yield: 8 servings

Nutritional Analysis: One (1 cup) serving equals 37 calories, 1 g fat 8 g carbohydrate, 1 g protein

Diabetic Exchanges: 1 vegetable

Soft Chicken Tacos

4 boneless skinless chicken breast halves (1 pound), cut into cubes

1 can (15 ounces) black beans, rinsed and drained

1 cup salsa

1 tablespoon taco seasoning

½ cup fat-free sour cream

6 low-carb, fat-free flour tortillas

Optional Toppings: shredded lettuce, fat-free shredded cheddar cheese, diced tomatoes, and sliced green onions.

In a skillet that has been coated with nonstick cooking spray, cook chicken until juices run clear. Add beans, salsa, and taco seasoning; heat through. Remove from heat and add sour cream. Spoon the chicken mixture down the center of each tortillas. Garnish with toppings of your choice.

Yield: 6 servings

Nutritional Analysis: One taco equals 196 calories, 4 g fat, 18 g carbohydrate, 22 g protein

Diabetic Exchanges: 1 starch, 2 lean meat

Spinach Chicken Wraps

1 package (10 ounces) fresh spinach

½ cup chopped fresh mushrooms

1 green onion, finely chopped

1 garlic cloves, minced

1 tablespoon olive oil

2 egg whites, lightly beaten

¼ cup crumbled feta cheese

¼ cup dry bread crumbs

¼ teaspoon dried rosemary, crushed

4 boneless skinless chicken breast halves (1 pound)

½ teaspoon dried basil

½ teaspoon dried thyme

¼ teaspoon pepper

4 low-carb, fat-free flour tortilla wraps

In a large saucepan, place spinach in a steamer basket over 1 in. of boiling water. Cover and steam for 2-3 minutes or just until wilted. When cool enough to handle, squeeze spinach dry and finely chop. In a nonstick skillet, sauté the mushrooms, onion, and garlic in oil until tender. Add spinach; cook and stir for 2 minutes. Transfer to a bowl. Add egg whites, cheese, and bread crumbs, mix well. Flatten chicken to ¼-in. thickness. Combine basil, thyme, and pepper; rub over one side of chicken. Spread spinach mixture over wraps and roll up. Secure with toothpicks. In a large saucepan, place wraps in a steamer basket over 1 in. of boiling water. Cover and steam for 12-15 minutes or until chicken is no longer pink.

Yield: 4 servings
Nutritional Analysis: One serving equals 238 calories, 6 g fat, 16 g carbohydrate, 30 g protein
Diabetic Exchanges: 2 lean meat, 1 vegetable, 1 fat

Broccoli Cheddar Soup

1 large bunch broccoli, coarsely chopped (5 cups)

2 tablespoons cornstarch

2 cups skim milk

1 cup chicken broth

1 tablespoon canola oil-based butter

¼ teaspoon salt

1/8 teaspoon pepper

1 cup (8 ounces) shredded fat-free cheddar cheese

Dash paprika

In a saucepan, bring 1 inch of water to a boil. Place broccoli in a steamer basket over water. Cover and steam for 5-8 minutes or until crisp-tender. Meanwhile, in another saucepan, combine the cornstarch, milk, and broth until smooth. Bring to a boil, cook, and stir for 2 minutes or until thickened.

Stir in the butter, salt, and pepper. Reduce heat. Add cheese and broccoli; heat just until cheese is melted. Sprinkle with paprika.

Yield: 4 servings

Nutritional Analysis: One serving equals 123 calories, 3 g fat, 17 g carbohydrate, 7 g protein

Diabetic Exchanges: 2 vegetable, 1 lean meat, 1 fat

BREAKFAST

Oat Waffles

1 cup all-purpose flour

1 cup oat flour

4 teaspoons baking powder

3 egg whites

1 ¾ cups skim milk

2 tablespoons canola oil

1 teaspoon vanilla extract

In a bowl, combine the first 3 ingredients. Combine the egg whites, milk, oil, and vanilla; stir into dry ingredients just until combined. Pour batter by ½ cupfuls into a preheated waffle iron; bake until golden brown.

Yield: 8 waffles

Nutritional Analysis: One waffle equals 147 calories, 3 g fat, 24 g carbohydrate, 6 g protein

Diabetic Exchanges: 1 ½ starch

Country Scrambled Eggs

12 egg whites, 2 yolks

¾ cup diced fully cooked ham

¾ cup fat-free shredded cheddar cheese

½ cup chopped fresh mushrooms

¼ cup chopped onion

In a bowl, beat eggs. Add ham, cheese, mushrooms, and onion. Lightly coat skillet with cooking spray; add egg mixture. Cook and stir over medium heat until eggs are completely set and cheese is melted.

Yield: 4 servings

Nutritional Analysis: One serving equals 134 calories, 6 g fat, 4 g carbohydrate, 16 g protein

Diabetic Exchanges: ½ vegetable, 1 fat, 1 ½ lean meats

Veggie Omelet

¼ cup diced green pepper

¼ cup diced onion

¼ cup sliced mushrooms

4 egg whites

Pinch pepper

2 tablespoons fat-free shredded cheddar cheese

In an 8-in. skillet, sauté green pepper, onion, and mushrooms in cooking spray until tender. Remove and set aside. In a small bowl, beat egg whites, salt, and pepper. Pour into a skillet. Cook over medium heat; as eggs set, lift edges, letting uncooked portion flow underneath. When the eggs are set, spoon vegetables and cheese over one side; fold omelet over filling. Cover and let stand for 1-2 minutes or until cheese is melted.

Yield: 1 serving

Nutritional Analysis: One serving equals 98 calories, 2 g fat, 3 g carbohydrate, 17 g protein

Diabetic Exchanges: 1 vegetable, 2 lean protein

Cheese Omelet

4 egg whites

¼ teaspoon onion powder

¼ teaspoon dried basil

¼ teaspoon dried parsley flakes

¼ cup fat-free shredded cheddar cheese

In a bowl, beat egg whites and seasonings. Lightly coat skillet with cooking spray. Add egg mixture; cook over medium heat. As eggs set, lift edges, letting uncooked portion flow underneath. When eggs are completely set, remove from the heat. Place cheese over half of the eggs. Fold in half and serve.

Yield: 1 serving

Nutritional Analysis: One serving equals 118 calories, 2 g fat, 6 g carbohydrate, 19 g protein

Diabetic Exchanges: 1 vegetable, 2 lean protein

Dilly Scrambled Eggs

6 egg whites, 2 yolks

¼ cup skim milk

1 teaspoon snipped fresh dill *or* ¼ teaspoon dill weed and dash of pepper

In a bowl, beat the eggs, milk, and pepper. Lightly coat skillet with cooking spray; add egg mixture. Cook and stir gently over medium heat until eggs are almost set. Sprinkle with cheese and dill; cook until eggs are completely set and cheese is melted.

Yield: 2 servings

Nutritional Analysis: One serving equals 139 calories, 7 g fat, 3 g carbohydrate, 16 g protein

Diabetic Exchanges: 1 fat, 2 lean protein

Spinach Egg Bake

1 cup seasoned bread crumbs

2 packages (10 ounces *each*) frozen chopped spinach, thawed and squeezed dry

3 cups (24 ounces) small-curd, fat-free cottage cheese

½ cup grated fat-free Parmesan cheese

8 egg whites, 2 yolks

Sprinkle ¼ cup bread crumbs into a cooking spray-coated 8-in. square baking dish. Bake at 350 degrees for 3-5 minutes or until golden brown. In a bowl, combine the spinach, cottage cheese, Parmesan cheese, six egg whites, one yolk, and remaining crumbs. Spread over the baked crumbs. Beat remaining eggs; pour over spinach mixture.

Bake uncovered at 350 degrees for 45 minutes or until a knife inserted near the center comes out clean. Let stand for 5-10 minutes before serving.

Yield: 4 servings

Nutritional Analysis: One serving equals 176 calories, 4 g fat, 15 g carbohydrate, 20 g protein

Diabetic Exchanges: 2 lean meat, 1 starch, 1 vegetable, 1 fat

DESSERTS

Creamy Raspberry Pie

1 package (3 ounces) sugar-free raspberry gelatin

½ cup boiling water

1 cup fat-free frozen vanilla yogurt

1 cup fresh *or* frozen unsweetened raspberries

¼ cup lime juice

2 cups fat-free whipped topping

1 reduced-fat graham cracker crust (9 inches)

Lime slices and additional raspberries and whipped topping, optional

In a bowl, dissolve the gelatin in boiling water. Stir in frozen yogurt until melted. Add raspberries and lime juice. Fold in whipped topping. Spoon into crust. Refrigerate for 3 hours or until firm. Garnish with lime, raspberries, and whipped topping.

Yield: 8 servings

Nutritional Analysis: One slice equals 86 calories, 2 g fat, 13 g carbohydrate, 4 g protein

Diabetic Exchanges: 1 starch, ½ fruit

Cherry Cream Pie

4 ounces fat-free cream cheese, softened

1 ½ cups sugar-free cherry pie filing

2 cups fat-free whipped topping

1 reduced-fat graham cracker crust (9 inches)

In a mixing bowl, beat cream cheese until smooth. Fold in the pie filling and whipped topping until blended. Spoon into crust. Cover and freeze for 8 hours or overnight. Remove from the freezer 15 minutes before serving.

Yield: 8 servings

Nutritional Analysis: One piece equals 94 calories, 2 g fat, 15 g carbohydrate, 4 g protein

Diabetic Exchanges: 1 starch, ½ fruit

Lemon Mousse

¼ cup sugar

Sugar substitute, such as Splenda or Stevia, equivalent to ½ cup sugar

½ cup cornstarch

3 cups skim milk

2/3 cup lemon juice

1 ½ teaspoons grated lemon peel

¼ teaspoon vanilla extract

2 cups fat-free whipped topping

In a saucepan, combine the sugar, sugar substitute, and cornstarch; gradually stir in milk until smooth. Bring to a boil over medium heat, stirring constantly. Cook and stir for 2 minutes or until thickened and bubbly. Remove from the heat. Stir in lemon juice, peel, and vanilla. Set saucepan in ice; stir until mixture reaches room temperature, about 5 minutes. Fold in whipped topping. Spoon into dessert dishes. Refrigerate for at least 1 hour before serving.

Yield: 10 servings

Nutritional Analysis: One (½ cup) serving equals 61 calories, 1 g fat, 10 g carbohydrate, 3 g protein

Diabetic Exchanges: 1 starch, 1 fruit

Pear Squares

1 ½ pounds pears, sliced

3 tablespoon all-purpose flour

¼ cup unsweetened apple juice concentrate

¾ cup reduced-fat graham cracker crumbs (about 10 squares)

½ teaspoon ground cinnamon

Dash ground nutmeg

2 tablespoons canola oil-based stick butter

½ cup fat-free whipped topping

Additional ground cinnamon

In a bowl, toss the pears, 1 tablespoon flour, and apple juice concentrate. Spoon into an 8-in. square baking dish coated with nonstick cooking spray. In a bowl, combine the crumbs, cinnamon, nutmeg, and remaining flour. Cut in butter until mixture resembles coarse crumbs. Sprinkle over pears.

Bake at 375 degrees for 30 minutes or until pears are tender and topping is lightly browned. Serve warm or chilled. Cut into squares; top with whipped topping and cinnamon.

Yield: 9 servings

Nutritional Analysis: One serving equals 128 calories, 4 g fat, 22 g carbohydrate, 1 g protein

Diabetic Exchanges: 1 starch, ½ fruit, ½ fat

Eggnog Pudding

2 cups skim milk

1 package (3.4 ounces) sugar-free instant vanilla pudding mix

½ teaspoon ground nutmeg

¼ teaspoon rum extract

Additional nutmeg, optional

In a bowl, combine the first 4 ingredients. Beat for 2 minutes. Spoon into individual dishes. Chill. Sprinkle with nutmeg if desired.

Yield: 4 servings

Nutritional Analysis: One (½ cup) serving equals 101 calories, 1 g fat, 16 g carbohydrate, 7 g protein.

Diabetic Exchanges: 1 starch, ½ lean meat

Orange Whip

1 can (11 ounces) mandarin oranges, drained

1 cup (8 ounces) fat-free, low-carb vanilla yogurt

2 tablespoons orange juice concentrate

2 cups fat-free whipped topping

In a bowl, combine the oranges, yogurt, and orange juice concentrate. Fold in the whipped topping. Spoon into serving dishes. Cover and freeze until firm. Remove from the freezer 20 minutes before serving.

Yield: 4 servings

Nutritional Analysis: One (¾ cup) serving equals 81 calories, 1 g fat, 15 g carbohydrate, 3 g protein

Diabetic Exchanges: 1 fruit, 1 starch

Blueberry Pie

¼ cup sugar

Sugar substitute, such as Splenda or Stevia, equivalent to ¼ cup sugar

2 tablespoons cornstarch

¾ cup water

4 cups fresh *or* frozen blueberries, thawed

1 reduced-fat graham cracker crust (9 inches)

Fat-free whipped topping

In a saucepan, combine sugar and cornstarch. Stir in water until smooth. Bring to a boil over medium heat, cook and stir for 2 minutes. Add blueberries. Cook for 3 minutes, stirring occasionally. Pour into crust. Chill. Garnish with whipped topping.

Yield: 8 servings

Nutritional Analysis: One piece equals 94 calories, 2 g fat, 17 g carbohydrate, 2 g protein

Diabetic Exchanges: 1 starch, 1 fruit

Light Carrot Cake

Sugar substitute equivalent to ¼ cup sugar

1 tablespoon canola oil

½ cup sugar-free apple sauce

1/3 cup orange juice concentrate

3 egg whites

1 cup all-purpose flour

1 teaspoon baking powder

1 teaspoon ground cinnamon

½ teaspoon ground allspice

¼ teaspoon baking soda

1 cup grated carrots

2 teaspoons confectioners' sugar

In a mixing bowl, combine the first 5 ingredients; beat for 30 seconds. Combine flour, baking powder, cinnamon, allspice, and baking soda; add to the orange juice mixture and mix well. Stir in carrots. Pour into an 8-in. square baking pan that has been coated with nonstick cooking spray. Bake at 350 degrees for 30 minutes or until a toothpick inserted near the center comes out clean. Cool; dust with confectioners' sugar.

Yield: 9 servings
Nutritional Analysis: One serving equals 147 calories, 3 g fat, 27 g carbohydrate, 3 g protein
Diabetic Exchanges: 2 starch, ½ fat

Chocolate Mousse

¾ cup skim milk

1 package (1.4 ounces) sugar-free instant chocolate pudding mix

½ cup fat-free sour cream

3 ounces fat-free cream cheese, cubed

½ teaspoon vanilla extract

1 carton (8 ounces) fat-free whipped topping

1 tablespoon chocolate cookie crumbs

In a bowl, whisk milk and pudding mix for 2 minutes (mixture will be very thick). In a mixing bowl, beat the sour cream, cream cheese, and vanilla. Add pudding; mix well. Fold in whipped topping. Spoon into individual dishes. Sprinkle with cookie crumbs. Refrigerate until serving.

Yield: 6 servings

Nutritional Analysis: One serving equals 106 calories, 2 g fat, 18 g carbohydrate, 4 g protein

Diabetic Exchanges: 1 ½ starch

Lemon Blueberry Cheesecake

1 package (3 ounces) sugar-free lemon gelatin

1 cup boiling water

2 tablespoons canola oil-based butter

1 tablespoon canola oil

1 cup reduced-fat graham cracker crumbs (about 16 squares)

1 carton (24 ounces) fat-free cottage cheese

¼ cup sugar

Sugar substitute equivalent to ¼ cup sugar

TOPPING:

Sugar substitute equivalent to 2 tablespoons sugar

1 ½ teaspoons cornstarch

¼ cup water

1 ½ cups fresh *or* frozen blueberries

1 teaspoon lemon juice

In a bowl, dissolve gelatin in boiling water; cool. Combine butter and oil; add crumbs and blend well. Press onto the bottom of a 9-in. springform pan. Chill. In a blender, process cottage cheese, sugar substitute, and sugar until smooth. While processing, slowly add cooled gelatin. Pour into crust; chill overnight.

For topping, combine sugar substitute and cornstarch in a saucepan; stir in water until smooth. Add 1 cup blueberries. Bring to a boil; cook and stir for 2 minutes or until thickened. Stir in lemon juice; cool slightly. Process in a blender until smooth. Refrigerate until completely cooled. Carefully run a knife around edge of pan to loosen cheesecake; remove sides of pan. Spread the blueberry mixture over the top. Top with remaining blueberries.

Yield: 12 servings
Nutritional Analysis: One piece equals 156 calories, 4 g fat, 22 g carbohydrate, 8 g protein
Diabetic Exchanges: 1 ½ starch, ½ fruit, ½ fat

No-Bake Chocolate Cheesecake

¾ cup reduced-fat graham cracker crumbs (about 12 squares)

2 tablespoons canola oil-based butter

1 envelope unflavored gelatin

1 cup cold water

4 squares (1 ounce *each*) semisweet chocolate, coarsely chopped

4 packages (8 ounces *each*) fat-free cream cheese

Sugar substitute equivalent to 1 cup sugar

¼ cup sugar

¼ cup baking cocoa

2 teaspoons vanilla extract

TOPPING:

2 cups fresh raspberries

1 ounce white candy coating

In a bowl, combine cracker crumbs and butter; press onto the bottom of a 9-in. spring form pan. Bake at 375 degrees for 8-10 minutes or until lightly browning. Cool on a wire rack.

For filling, in a small saucepan, sprinkle gelatin over cold water; let stand for 1 minute. Heat over low heat, stirring until gelatin is completely dissolved. Add the semisweet chocolate; stir until melted. In a mixing bowl, beat the cream cheese, sugar substitute, and sugar until smooth. Gradually add the chocolate mixture and cocoa. Beat in vanilla. Pour into crust; refrigerate for 2-3 hours or until firm. Arrange raspberries on top of cheesecake. In a heavy saucepan or microwave, melt white candy coating; stir until smooth. Drizzle or pipe over berries. Carefully run a knife around edge of pan to loosen. Remove sides of pan.

Yield: 12 servings

Nutritional Analysis: One slice equals 158 calories, 6 g fat, 27 g carbohydrate, 9 g protein

Diabetic Exchanges: 2 starch, 1 lean meat, 1 fat

Pumpkin Spice Dip

1 package (8 ounces) fat-free cream cheese

½ cup canned pumpkin

Sugar substitute equivalent to ½ cup sugar

1 teaspoon ground cinnamon

1 teaspoon vanilla extract

1 teaspoon maple flavoring

½ teaspoon pumpkin pie spice

½ teaspoon ground nutmeg

1 carton (8 ounces) fat-free whipped topping

In a large mixing bowl, combine the cream cheese, pumpkin, and sugar substitute; mix well. Beat in the cinnamon, vanilla, maple flavoring, pumpkin pie spice, and nutmeg. Fold in whipped topping. Refrigerate until serving.

Yield: 4 cups

Nutritional Analysis: One serving (3 tablespoons) equals 33 calories, 1 g fat, 4 g carbohydrate, 1 g protein

Diabetic Exchanges: ½ starch

Peanut Butter Pudding

2 cups skim milk

4 tablespoons reduced-fat creamy peanut butter

1 package (1 ounce) sugar-free instant vanilla pudding mix

½ cup fat-free whipped topping

4 teaspoons chocolate syrup

In a bowl, whisk the milk and peanut butter until blended. Add pudding mix, whisk for 2 minutes or until slightly thickened. Spoon into dessert dishes. Refrigerate for at least 5 minutes or until set. Just before serving, dollop with shipped topping and drizzle with chocolate syrup.

Yield: 4 servings

Nutritional Analysis: One serving equals 172 calories, 8 g fat, 17 g carbohydrate, 8 g protein

Diabetic Exchanges: 1 starch, 1 lean meat, 1 fat

CHAPTER EIGHT KEY POINTS

1) The right foods in the right amounts should be your focus.

2) You can construct fancy recipes, but this is unnecessary. Be creative and plan ahead using foods you like.

3) Did I mention "be creative"?

Chapter Nine

PUTTING IT ALL TOGETHER

Come on, Doc, Does it Really Work?

You can take the most important step to ensure your success right now. When a client leaves my office for the first time, I can predict his or her success with indescribable accuracy. I observe people interacting with science and life. I see people succeed, and I see people fail. The best and most accurate information means nothing if you don't or can't apply it. My clients who take the initiative never fail. This first step is critical: it is simply to start now. Use the Six Week Program Guide (or your own notebook) and start recording your food intake now. Waiting until tomorrow will lead you to next week; next week will lead you to failure, and you may just throw away your last chance to gain total control over food, your health, and your physique. Start today. Sound like a broken record yet? Record everything you eat for a day or two as you make small changes that you easily recall from this book. Start fine-tuning your nutrition by making better-quality food choices, improving your meal spacing, concentrating on meal ratios, and reaching your target personal Diet Doc Rx. Before you know it, you'll be feeling better than you thought possible, losing weight, and you'll be well on your way to becoming your own nutritionist.

Guaranteed?

It's hard for me not to guarantee success to everyone, because I know that success is possible if you follow the program. The greatest deterrent to your achievement once you get started is reaching too high a comfort level too soon. I occasionally have a client who starts with the incredible motivation that comes with the new understanding of nutrition. He or she starts losing two to three pounds a week, refers friends to our facility, and is overjoyed with the results. This client meticulously documents food and nutrient totals and consistently

Stress Eating is the Real Deal

You've heard the commercials for cortisol-reducing supplements. "Block the hormone that traps unwanted fat around your stomach..." I'm not sure if the supplements can do much to stop your adrenal glands from producing cortisol, but a valid point is raised. Many of us admittedly are "stress eaters" or "emotional eaters." There is a very good reason. Under stress, and your brain doesn't care if it's from being chased by a grizzly bear, deadlines at work, or watching the nightly news, your body goes into "fight of flight" response. Your heart rate increases, blood is shunted to your muscles for action, and stored carbohydrates (glycogen) are diverted from your liver and muscle into your bloodstream for the anticipated energy needs.

As the process slows – assuming you didn't get caught by the bear or your boss – that extra blood glucose gets stored as abdominal fat. It is directed mainly to your middle because only there can it be mobilized rapidly again for conversion to glucose. Your body is thinking ahead – for survival. The problem is we're getting more and more chronic daily stress and we're not using the released energy. It gets worse.

The storage of the new fat deposits signal the brain to shut off the stress response and the next phase of fight or flight is launched: operation refuel. The hard-wired expectancy of the nervous system is that after a stressful situation, energy will have to be replaced. Waves of cravings follow as part of the let-down from stress. Cortisol not only causes direct abdominal fat storage but intense carbohydrate cravings. (Just a side note: many researchers now directly link antidepressant drugs to obesity for this same reason. Apparently, we get locked into this step that involves bringing stress levels down when we take these medications.) Stress must be met head on with preparedness. When our daily lives create turmoil and intense hunger follows, you can combat it by relaxing, performing breathing exercises, walking away from the situation, drinking a glass of water, etc. This is to literally buy yourself time and direct your brain to de-escalate the situation. If you find yourself reaching for food, realize the situation at hand and make sure it doesn't lead to a binge. With this information you don't have to be dragged under the tow of this hormone; you can stay on top with planning.

progresses. Then one day, progress slows; sometimes this person starts regaining weight. All of a sudden, either "it's just not working anymore" or they suddenly "have a slow metabolism." I ask to see their nutrition journal, and the reply is often, "Well, I quit writing things down last month." Translation: "I've lost my motivation. I'm cheating. In short, I'm no longer doing what needs to be done."

As soon as this client gets back on track – guess what? Their results pick right up where they left off. The point of this drawn-out example is that you must be consistent to reach your goal. It is so easy to slip upward into "maintenance" eating. You're still eating perhaps the right percentages of macronutrients, but add just a little too much food and the intake volume may take you out of the losing range and into the maintenance range. My advice would be to stick with your weight-loss level of food intake for as long as you can and then take a planned break where you increase your volume to a maintenance level to "catch your breath," regroup, and then go right back to progressing. I can't emphasize enough that your initial progress and understanding needs to be underlined by consistency.

Prepare to Win!

Once you've gotten off to a great start, prepare for a long journey of experimentation, changes, new understanding, and better integration of proper nutrition into your daily life. A shift in your thought processes regarding food has to occur. It is incredibly rewarding for me to see a client lose the 34th and 35th pounds, or to have a client reach the goal of losing 15 pounds in 8 weeks. However, I'm ecstatic when I see that client enjoying a higher quality of life a year later – without having gained any weight back. This long-term success has very little to do with me. I take great pleasure in knowing that clients took the right information and worked consistently hard to win what were perhaps great wars in their lives. I can educate and motivate, but ultimately it's you that will or will not succeed. We may all fall down once in awhile, but unfortunately not all of us will get back up. As the initial motivation wears off and the ice cream is no longer as easy to pass up, you have to remember who you're doing this for. You now have the tools to pick yourself up. You have a plan that's a proven success; you're no longer stumbling around in the dark. I know you can do it!

CHAPTER NINE KEY POINTS

▸ 1) Start right now!

▸ 2) Document meticulously.

▸ 3) Consistency, consistency, consistency.

▸ 4) It doesn't matter how many times you fall down, only how many times you get back up!

▸ 5) You're in this for life – be patient and enjoy the trip!

▸ 6) Prepare your mind for battle; prepare to win!!

Chapter Ten

SIX WEEK METABOLIC TRANSFORMATION

Let's Get Started!!

I have seen a lot of "eureka" moments over my career as clients start to understand past errors and connect the dots of sound nutrition. Rarely does a client leave without thinking they've found the missing link, excited to begin their new program. Rarely, however, do they start without getting overwhelmed by the sheer volume of new information. This six-week start is an incredible tool that will cement all the physiology you find on these pages into your eating habits – one step at a time! Following this six-week program has become as close to a 100% guarantee for your success as anything I have ever seen.

Week One

Week one has a single focus. I want you to get familiar with the charting system provided and begin the process of tracking your food intake. This week may be frustrating as you start measuring food, planning meals, and calculating nutrients for journaling. The rare person who fails often stops here. If you're committed to your goals, you'll survive this step and will have ensured your success. Take this week very seriously, and you'll understand why I feel it's the most critical. Once you go through the learning process of tracking your food, you'll have a literal databank of nutritional information memorized without even trying! As you look up foods, read nutrition fact panels, scour menus, and record your intake, you'll be amazed how easy it becomes.

At the end of the first week, you should be getting into your personal Rx ranges consistently. The first couple days will be hit and miss; don't expect yourself to be perfect. This week is a learning process to help you to understand the documentation and slowly get used to what those suggested protein, carbohydrate, and fat intake ranges mean in terms of real food. It's one thing to see numbers on paper and another to translate them into meals!

It may be a good idea to keep your personal Diet Doc Rx card, which I provided at the back of the book, in your pocket or in your nutrition journal. Jot down the food counts for meals you frequently eat. That way you don't have to calculate them over and over and can make faster decisions on the spot.

At the end of this chapter, there is a sample daily food chart and a six-week "at-a-glance" spreadsheet. Record the all-important daily food, amounts, and times on a form similar to this. It will help you keep a running tally and in planning for the rest of the day. The weekly chart is a great tool to study trends and really zero in on what levels of food intake allow for different weight-loss paces. Without this objectivity you may find yourself going nowhere fast.

Week One Steps to Success:

1) Record your beginning weight, body composition measurements (if you're having a professional monitor your body fat percentage), and your suggested nutrient intake totals.

2) Plan a sample day by creating meals that include quality foods as discussed in the book, meal volumes that are appropriate, meal times that fit in your schedule, and adjust the meal amounts until the total amount of protein, carbohydrates, and fat fall into your suggested ranges at the end of the day.

3) Plan ahead for the day and make sure you have the food available that you'll need.

4) Record food intake throughout the day.

5) Make adjustments for the next day if necessary; remember, this is the first week and you shouldn't be perfect yet!

6) At the end of the week weigh yourself. (Keep in mind that losing more than one to two pounds will initially be water loss.)

7) Review your week and focus on "lessons learned" so you can improve for next week.

8) Keep your Diet Docs' Rx card with you for quick reference.

Week Two

Hopefully you now agree that going through week one with diligence was critical to your success. Now you have a great base of experience to know what all those grams of protein, carbohydrates, and fat really mean in a day of food intake. Week two's objective is to refine your meals and work on making sure your program is going to be perfect for you, individually. Chapter three offered guidance in creating meals that would be fairly consistent in volume, timing, and quality so that your food will be properly consumed throughout the day. Recall that blood chemistry stability is a major factor in how you'll feel and how effective your weight loss will be. I want you to experience more energy than you thought possible and minimize your hunger. This is easily accomplished by focusing on the "nuts and bolts" of your food throughout the day.

First, this week will be a fair assessment of the amount of food you're consuming. The first week's weight loss was a combination of water loss and fat loss, but this week will allow a better look at actual fat loss. Two to three pounds for men and one to two pounds for women is about perfect. Faster loss may indicate that you're in danger of losing muscle, getting too hungry, and being prone to overeating. Review chapter two on how to adjust your nutrient numbers if you're losing too fast or too slowly.

Glance back through your first week's journal of your food intake. Check for the consistency of your daily numbers, spacing between meals, and meal volume. Are you too high or too low on protein, carbs, or fat? Were there some large gaps between meals (four hours or more)? I disagree with nutritionists who try to get people to have the exact same ratios and amounts of food at exact time intervals, but for all the reasons I discussed in chapter three, there has to be some consistency. The amount of flexibility I feel is appropriate is for your own hunger patterns and for schedule normalcy. It can be a scheduling issue as to when you can eat a whole-food meal and when you may need a protein bar or shake. These are elements for you to decide based on your social situation and based on your hunger, likes, and dislikes. If, however, you aren't seeing the results you want, you may have to revisit this step and make sure you're not sabotaging your progress out of convenience. I want to make things as easy as possible, but some foods may need to be sacrificed for you to progress.

Week Two Steps to Success:

1) Review your first week of journaling. Look at daily nutrient totals, meal spacing, and recall subjective thoughts such as hunger, energy level, and ease of meal consumption.

2) Alter your meal plans if necessary due to schedule inconvenience or hunger patterns. Experiment to see if you can improve for your own comfort level.

3) Purposely increase your variety of foods to expand your arsenal of potential meals and snacks.

4) Start journaling subjective comments so you can relate your body's response to what you're consuming.

5) Weigh yourself and determine if you're losing too fast or too slow. Adjust your program according to chapter two.

Week Three

Now you're on your way to permanent success. Whether you realize it or not, you have altered your eating habits and have gained a great deal of invaluable knowledge by hanging in this long. You have fine-tuned your food volume for a typical day which will satisfy proper nutritional needs to lose body fat and maintain lean body mass. If you're losing too fast or too slow, keep adjusting your totals based on the information in chapter two. Excellent documentation of your nutrition is key to making sure you have as objective a guide as possible.

It's time to look at the details of the actual food you're consuming. This would be a good time to review chapter four and increase your understanding of carbohydrates. When you're dieting, the glycemic index, carbohydrate volume per meal, and avoiding sugar and trigger foods becomes paramount. You want little rolling insulin fluctuations in your bloodstream, not mountainous spikes.

Carbohydrates, I must repeat, are the body's primary energy source. At this point in your program, you may feel some hunger return if you're generally not eating enough calories. Most people believe they are eating more food than normal just because of the increase in protein and fibrous carbohydrates and because power spacing helps them feel full. However, it's also a common pattern for people to start letting protein levels slide and start increasing carbohydrate intake again. If you are heading in this direction, it's a slow path back to a plateau. Keep your carbs in check because too much carbohydrate intake will block your body's need to use an alternative energy source – body fat.

Recall that blood chemistry stability is a great focus. Make sure you're not elevating carbohydrates too high at meals or leaving gaping holes in your day without enough. Look at your food journaling and make sure you have some balance in your meals and snacks. They don't have to be exact replicas of each other, but you should avoid major inconsistencies as you seek to end up within your carbohydrate range for the day. Too many in one meal and you'll end up lethargic and then very hungry. Too few for too many hours and you will also end up hungry and unable to pull in the reigns at the kitchen table.

Week Three Steps to Success:

1) Review chapter four regarding carbohydrates.

2) Review your daily nutrition intake and take steps to make sure it's consistent daily.

3) Use a good measure of balance in your carbohydrate intake meal to meal. Avoid too much in meals and avoid allowing too much time between meals.

4) Start paying close attention to the glycemic index and note which carb sources trigger hunger a short while after the meal and which ones delay hunger.

5) Weigh yourself and adjust your nutrient intake as described in chapter two if necessary.

Week Four

I like to view fat as a variable, second only to carbohydrates, that can be used to sustain body fat loss if manipulated correctly. Chapter five provides plenty of detail regarding the function of fat in the body and the differences between "good" and "bad" fat. The practical application of fat can be simplified. Once you have created some good habits, including the addition of some healthy unsaturated fats, you'll have to cut the saturated fats to a minimum to stay within your daily range. If fat intake is as moderate as I suggest and healthy fats are the dominant source, then dietary fat will never take the blame for lack of progress. However, if the table starts tilting toward an increased fat intake (especially with a higher inclusion of saturated fats), a cascade of events will take place. First, the calorie-rich fat may take you right up to a maintenance range of food intake from your planned calorie deficit. This is common in people who mistakenly think carbs are the only thing to worry about. A hefty handful of almonds may seem like the best thing to eat to avoid letting the carbs get too high, but if the extra fat increases the total calories for the day out of a deficit range, a day of fat loss is missed. Portion size and daily food volume are critical steps.

Second, fat can be absorbed straight from the bloodstream and into your fat cells. Too much fat in a meal on a day in which calories weren't low enough results in a lack of progress and may actually lead to regaining a small amount of fat. Excessive amounts of fat can only be used as energy successfully if carbs are near zero, such as in a ketogenic diet. As previously discussed, however, this isn't the best or easiest way to lose weight. Make sure you're not letting your dietary fat grams climb if you mistakenly tend to focus only on carbs.

The bottom line is to make sure you include a variety of healthy unsaturated fats wherever you can in your diet. Keep fat sources spaced evenly throughout the day. Spacing will make it easier to stay in your suggested totals, allowing for slower digestion and better maintenance of blood glucose levels. More importantly, it helps keep hunger in check.

Week Four Steps to Success:

1) Pick a variety of unsaturated fats that can be used as at least 50% of your fat intake.

2) Space fat intake as evenly as possible within meal structure.

3) Don't let fat intake creep up just to keep carbs down.

4) Perform your weekly review of nutrition journaling for consistency and check your body weight for progress. Make your best effort to correct problem areas in carrying out your program and adjust your program according to chapter two if necessary.

Week Five

Minimizing protein's role in weight loss would be a mistake. As a matter of fact, behaviorally it is one of the best indicators of a client's success. I won't repeat the body's utilization of amino acids for cell function (I don't want you to fall asleep and start drooling on your new Diet Doc book). I'll stick instead to what will help you lose and control weight permanently. Most who embark upon this journey will have to raise their protein to a level they're not used to. I certainly don't advocate unsafe or unhealthy levels, but most of us just don't eat enough. Basal metabolic function requires approximately 50 to 70 grams of protein a day just to stay in "neutral," and that doesn't account for the potential increased needs to do the calorie deficit of dieting and exercise.

When protein is consumed, it is digested slowly. Other foods eaten at the same time are therefore digested and absorbed slowly as well. After those meals, blood chemistry will be more stable for a longer period. Hunger will be lower and energy will be higher. You don't have to eat protein at every meal, but there are some key times. Breakfast is a good place to eat some protein to prevent hunger shortly thereafter. If you can't eat much protein at breakfast, make sure you get some in your first snack such as a protein bar or shake. Dinner is also a meal in which you want to have a whole-food protein source to help prevent late evening hunger. These suggestions are based on years of experience as to what can help you succeed, but should be coupled with your own personal observations of your hunger patterns and schedule preferences.

The practical side of protein that I mentioned in the first paragraph relates heavily to hunger. It may have taken you a week or two to get your protein levels up to your suggested ranges. While weight loss is steady and energy is increasing, it is easy to ride this high just because of the positive reinforcement. But eventually, the rigors of daily life start competing with that momentum and it's easier to make choices due to convenience instead of conviction. Protein intake starts decreasing, hunger therefore increases, and reflexively, carbohydrate consumption increases again. Voila: the recipe for slipping out of a body fat burning mode. I work with a lot of professional bodybuilders, and I have to tell you that what works for them will work for us. When fat has to come off, eating enough protein absolves hunger, creates a more fat-loss-friendly internal environment, and just pulls a lot of things into place. I automatically lose weight faster when I include a protein shake or two as snacks. They keep blood sugar stable, cut cravings, and save more fat and carbs for meals. You can eat a whole-food protein source as a snack as well, but when you find it difficult to get enough protein, remember to choose habits that are easy to maintain.

		Week Five Steps to Success:
1)		Make sure protein levels aren't sliding downward.
2)		Keep protein sources lean whenever possible. Save fattier selections for occasional meals.
3)		Consider protein bars or shakes for snacks if protein levels are difficult to achieve.
4)		Review your charting and look for a link between lower-protein days and increased hunger and possible increases in carb intake.
5)		Unwanted hunger often is preceded by low-protein meals. Consider increasing protein at those meals.
6)		Check body weight for progress and adjust nutrient numbers per chapter two if necessary.

Week Six

You're now coasting through the middle portion of your weight-loss program. Reviewing all the key points in this six-week program from time to time will help keep the driving principles in the forefront of your mind. You may also consider reading certain chapters again for additional assessment of your progress. Week 6 is dedicated to an evaluation of your progress and a management plan for the rest of your time in weight-loss mode which may be another 3, 6, or 18 months. After that, you'll arrive at the incredible day of being able to celebrate the success of reaching your goal and increasing your food toward maintenance levels!

Before we get there, however, let's keep our hands on the plow and make sure we have the good fortune of reaching that point. Look at your daily charting of protein, carbohydrate, and fat intake. Carefully compare that information to your weight-loss progress. Pay attention even to overall calorie intake. Calculate weekly averages for those statistics and look for the relationship between the level of food and macronutrients you're eating and your rate of weight loss. You should be able to see a causal relationship between the two. You can observe with clarity and precision how much food you can eat each day (on average) and lose one pound, two pounds, or whatever your healthy desired rate, based on these records. Now you may see one reason I dictate that this documentation is key to your success. You have created a database that will enable you to manage your weight control for as long as you wish.

That is exactly our goal for the remainder of your program. Decide what pace you would like to continue (based on our recommendations of safe weight loss and your own comfort level), and plan meals and daily nutritional totals accordingly. Keep monitoring your progress and recording your food intake as you add to your knowledge. Understand that there will be an occasional setback or a social situation at which you anticipate not "eating perfectly" according to your plan, but if these are infrequent, you'll see your progress continue.

Week Six Steps to Success:

1) *Review weekly weight-loss rate and compare with weekly averages of all three macronutrients.*

2) *Compare the relationship of this data for accurate estimations of the food intake required for different rates of weekly weight loss.*

3) *Celebrate the completion of your first six weeks!! (Yahooooooo!)*

NUTRITION JOURNAL

DATE: _____ WEEK: _____ DAY: _____ WEIGHT: _____

MEAL	PORTION SIZE	FOOD CONSUMED	TOTAL GRAMS PER MEAL			CALORIES
			Pro	Carb	Fat	
1						
2						
3						
4						
5						
6						
7						
TOTALS FOR DAY						

Monthly Nutrition Log

Week One

Day	Protein	Carbs	Fat	Calories	Comments	Weight
1						
2						
3						
4						
5						
6						
7						
Averages						

Week Two

Day	Protein	Carbs	Fat	Calories	Comments	Weight
1						
2						
3						
4						
5						
6						
7						
Averages						

Week Three

Day	Protein	Carbs	Fat	Calories	Comments	Weight
1						
2						
3						
4						
5						
6						
7						
Averages						

Monthly Nutrition Log

Week Four

Day	Protein	Carbs	Fat	Calories	Comments	Weight
1						
2						
3						
4						
5						
6						
7						
Averages						

Week Five

Day	Protein	Carbs	Fat	Calories	Comments	Weight
1						
2						
3						
4						
5						
6						
7						
Averages						

Week Six

Day	Protein	Carbs	Fat	Calories	Comments	Weight
1						
2						
3						
4						
5						
6						
7						
Averages						

Chapter Eleven

KEEP IT OFF FOREVER!

There would be nothing more disheartening than to gain back a significant portion of the weight you lost once you've worked so hard for so long. You may already know exactly what I'm talking about from past experience. You can stop this pattern if you take this transition seriously.

Some of the blame for this misfortune lies, again, at the foot of physiology. The habits created when dieting and the excitement of success held you to your previous diet. However, if that plan included a severe decrease in carbohydrates or insufficient calories, your metabolic rate may have suffered significantly. Once a higher food intake is reestablished, you may have regained body fat rapidly until your metabolic rate rebounded. By then, it was too late. That is the danger of a very low-calorie or low-carb diet.

A second reason for failure, and often in conjunction with the first, is letting your guard down and not adjusting your food properly. If you were to charge through a few days of really high-carb intake, especially the typical binge or "celebration" foods, it is very hard to recover. The wildly fluctuating blood sugar will spin you into levels of hunger you aren't used to. Before you know it, you're eating an incredible amount of carbohydrates and converting a large portion of them into body fat again. This is the exact cycle you bought this book to avoid.

Once you have reached your goal, you have to bring your food intake up to a maintenance level where you will no longer be losing, but, of course, not gaining. You will not have to raise your protein levels; they have already been set to give you an ideal amount. Your fat and carbohydrates may be raised in tandem but not necessarily in equal amounts. You may find that 10 to 15 extra grams of fat and 25 grams of carbs will provide enough energy and calories as the first step toward raising your food intake to a maintenance level. This may slow your rate of loss, but not stop it completely. Take another step upward, and then another.

Many important things will happen if you make this process incremental. First, your blood chemistry will remain more stable and you'll be less likely to experience binge-causing hunger due to the increase in carbohydrates. Second, you'll slowly rebuild any decreases in your metabolic rate that may have occurred due to the length of your diet. This will ensure that you won't regain body fat at all. As a matter of fact, you'll find you have to slowly keep adding more food to not lose weight! The amount of carbohydrates and fat that you add is entirely up to you, but keep several health and behavioral points in mind.

You still want to adhere to the same health-building habits that you created along the way. Keep good fats in your diet and keep saturated fats low. Stick with low-glycemic index carbs as much as you can (for all the reasons you dieted with them). If you can maintain most of these principles, your increase in food will leave you with high energy, stability, and controlled weight. Experiment with different levels of carbohydrates and fat at your decided maintenance level of food. You may find that you feel and "operate" better with one macronutrient raised disproportionately to the other. This has to do with metabolic body type. An insulin-sensitive person may get hungrier on a higher level of carbs and tend to gain weight back. However, with carbs remaining a little lower and fat increasing, the same person may have no hunger, high energy, and no weight gain. A person fortunate enough to have a high metabolism tends to be an "ectomorph" and be able to consume a higher percentage of calories from carbs without weight gain. Beware, though, despite being able to get away with more carbs, an ectomorph can still gain weight.

One last point: as you transition into maintenance, you are leaving a dieting level of food that includes less carbs than your body needs for energy. As you increase your food, you will be refilling your liver and muscles with a higher amount of glycogen. Glycogen attracts and holds water. You will undoubtedly gain a couple of pounds due to that fact just as the first couple of lost pounds were water. Don't be alarmed; this is normal hydration and a normal level of carbohydrates stored in your body. You just want to make sure you don't gain more than a couple pounds back once you've hit your lowest weight. Your body fat level won't be affected; the weight will be just water and glycogen. This is another reason to keep your upward changes slow and incremental. You don't want to fret over water gain, but you also don't want to be deceived into thinking that you're gaining just water when it may be fat.

So, there you have it. If patiently and scientifically handled, the transition into maintenance can be smooth and successful. Instead of regain, you can have an increasing level of energy, an increasing metabolic rate, and control of your weight. That, after all, is my goal for you.

The Diet Doc Rx

- Document everything.
- Only one "splurge" meal per week (not a day or a weekend or...).
- Eat five to six times per day (three meals and two to three snacks).
- Eat even if you don't feel hungry initially to prevent bingeing ("stay ahead of hunger").
- Weigh/measure your food initially (make sure an ounce is an ounce, a cup is a cup...).
- Read labels carefully and watch portion size.
- Exercise five to six times per week and try to strength train at least two of those days.
- Keep constantly armed with good foods.

My Personal Rx (grams/day)

Protein _____

Carbs _____

Fat _____

BIBLIOGRAPHY

Abbasi, F., et al. 2000. "High carbohydrate diets, triglyceride rich lipoproteins, and coronary heart disease risk." *American Journal of Cardiology* 85:45-48.

Acheson, K.J., et al. 1984. "Nutritional influences on lipogenesis and thermogenesis after a carbohydrate meal." *American Journal of Physiology* 246:E62-E70.

Agus, M.S.D., et al. 2000. "Dietary composition and physiologic adaptations to energy restriction." *American Journal of Clinical Nutrition* 71:901-7.

Ascherio, A., and W.C. Willet. 1997. "Health effects of transfatty acids." *American Journal of Clinical Nutrition* 66:1006S-1010S.

Atkins, R.C. 2002. *Dr. Atkins' New Diet Revolution.* Avon, New York, NY.

Baba, N.H., et al. 1999. "High protein versus high carbohydrate hypoenergetic diet for the treatment of obese hyperinsulinemic subjects." *International Journal of Obesity* 11:1202-1206.

Brand-Miller, J.C. et al. 2002. "Glycemic index and obesity." *American Journal of Clinical Nutrition* 76:281S-285S.

Brand-Miller, J., et al. 2003. *The New Glucose Revolution.* Marlowe and Company, New York, NY.

Bravata, D.M., L. Sanders, J. Huang, et al. 2003. "Efficacy and safety of low-carbohydrate diets: a systematic review." *Journal of the American Medical Association* 289;14:1837-1850.

Bray, G.A. 1969. "Effect of caloric restrictions on energy expenditure in obese patients." *Lancet* 2:397-8.

Bray, G.A. 2003. "Low-carbohydrate diets and realities of weight loss." *Journal of the American Medical Association* 289;14:1853-1855.

Brody, T. 1999. *Nutritional Biochemistry,* Second ed. Academic Press, San Diego, CA.

Brownell, K.D., M.R.C. Greenwood, E. Stellar, and E.E. Shrager. 1986. "The effects of repeated cycles of weight loss and regain in rats." *Physiology Behavior* 38:459-64.

Campfield, L., F. Smith, and P. Burn. 1998. "Strategies and potential molecular targets for obesity treatment." *Science* 280:1383-1387.

Carlola, R., J.P. Harley, and C.R. Noback. 1990. *Human Anatomy and Physiology.* McGraw-Hill, New York, NY.

Chinachoti, P. 1995. "Carbohydrates: Functionality in foods." *American Journal of Clinical Nutrition* 61:922S-929S.

Clark, L.T., K.C. Ferdinand, and D.P. Ferdinand. 2003. *Contemporary Management of the Metabolic Syndrome.* McMahon Publishing Group, New York, NY.

Crapo, P.A. 1985. "Simple versus complex carbohydrate use in the diabetic diet." *Annual Review of Nutrition* 5:95-114.

Daly, M.E. et al. 1997. "Dietary carbohydrate and insulin sensitivity: A review of the evidence and clinical implications." *American Journal of Clinical Nutrition* 66:1072-1085.

Depres, J.P., et al. 1996. "Hyperinsulinemia as an independent risk factor for ischemic heart disease." *New England Journal of Medicine* 334:952-957.

Dune, L.J. 1990. *Nutrition Almanac*, 3rd ed. McGraw-Hill, New York, NY.

Eades, M.R. and M.D. Eades. 1996. *Protein Power.* Bantam Books, New York, NY.

Ely, D.L. 1997. "Overview of dietary sodium effects on and interactions with cardiovascular and neuroendocrine functions." *American Journal of Clinical Nutrition* 65:594S-605S.

Erikson, R.H. and Y.S. Kim. 1990. "Digestion and absorption of dietary protein." *Annual Review of Medicine* 41:133-139.

Felig, P., et al. 1970. "Amino acid metabolism in the regulation of gluconeogenesis in man." *American Journal of Clinical Nutrition* 23:986-992.

Felig, P., J.D. Baxter, and L.A. Frohman. 1995. *Endocrinology and Metabolism,* 3rd ed. McGraw-Hill, New York, NY.

Figlewicz, D.P., et al. 1996. "Endocrine regulation of food intake and body weight." *Journal of Laboratory and Clinical Medicine* 127:328-332.

Fisler, J.S., et al. 1982. "Nitrogen economy during very low calorie reducing diets." *American Journal of Clinical Nutrition* 35:471-486.

Flegal, K.M., B.I. Graubard, D.F. Williamson, and M.H. Gail. 2005. "Excess deaths associated with underweight, overweight, and obesity." *Journal of the American Medical Association* 293;15:1861-68.

Ford, E.S., and S.Liu. 2001. "Glycemic index and serum high-density-lipoprotein cholesterol concentration among US adults." *Archives of Internal Medicine* 161:572-48.

Fordslund, A.H., et al. 1999. "Effect of protein intake and physical activity on twenty-four hour pattern and rate of micronutrient utilization." *American Physiology Society* E964-E976.

Foster-Powell, K., J.C. Brand-Miller, S.H.A. Holt. 2002. "International table of glycemic index and glycemic load values: 2002." *American Journal of Clinical Nutrition* 76:5-56.

Fraser, G.E., J. Sabate, W.L. Beeson, and T.M. Strahan.. 1992. "A Possible Protective Effect of Nutrition Consumption on Risk of Coronary Heart Disease—The Adventist Health Study." *Archives of Internal Medicine* 152:1416-1424.

Friedman, H.I. and B. Nylund. 1980. "Intestinal fat digestion, absorption, and transport." *American Journal of Clinical Nutrition* 33:1108-1139.

Frost, G. and A. Dornhorst. 2000. "The relevance of the glycemic index to our understanding of dietary carbohydrates." *Diabetic Medicine* 17:336-45

Fushiki, T., et al. 1989. "Changes in glucose transporters in muscle in response to glucose." *American Journal of Physiology* 256:E580-E587.

Golay, A., et al. 1996. "Weight loss with low or high carbohydrate diet?" *International Journal of Obesity and Related Metabolic Disorders* 20:1067-1072.

Goldman, L. and J.C. Bennett. 2000. *Cecil Textbook of Medicine* 21st ed. Saunders, Philadelphia, PA.

Gottfried, S.S. 1993. *Biology Today.* Mosby, St. Louis, MO.

Groff, J.L. and S.S. Gropper. 2000. *Advanced Nutrition and Human Metabolism.* Wadsworth Thomson Learning, Stamford, CT.

Gross, L.S., E.S. Ford, and S. Liu. 2004. "Increased consumption of refined carbohydrates and the epidemic of type 2 diabetes in the United States:an ecologic assessment." American *Journal of Clinical Nutrition.*79:774-9.

Holloszy, J. and W. Kohrt. 1996. "Regulation of carbohydrate and fat metabolism during and after exercise." *Annual Review of Nutrition* 16:121-138.

Holman, R.T. 1988. "George O. Burr and the discovery of essential fatty acids." *Journal of Nutrition* 118:535-540.

Hu, F.B., W.C. Willett, T. Li, et al. 2004. "Adiposity as compared with physical activity in predicting mortality among women." *New England Journal of Medicine* 351:2694-703.

Hudgins, L., et al. 2000. "Relationship between carbohydrate induced hypertriglyceridemia and fatty acid synthesis in lean and obese subjects." *Journal of Lipid Research* 41:595-604.

Jenkins, D.J., C.W. Kendall, A. Marchie, and L.S. Augustin. 2004. "Too much sugar, too much carbohydrate, or just too much?" *American Journal of Clinical Nutriton* 79:711-2.

Leaf, A. and P.C. Weber. 1988. "Cardiovascular effects of n-3 fatty acids." *New England Journal of Medicine* 318:549-557.

Leeds, A.R. 2002. "Glycemic index and heart disease." *American Journal of Clinical Nutrition* 76:286S-289S.

Leibel, R.L., M. Rosenbaum, and J. Hirsch. 1995. "Changes in energy expenditure resulting from altered body weight." *New England Journal of Medicine* 332:621-628.

Leibowitz, S.F. 1992. "Neurochemical-neuroendocrine systems in the brain controlling macronutrient intake and metabolism." *Trends in Neuroscience* 15:491-497.

Liu, Simmin, W.C. Willett, J.E. Manson, et al. 2003. Relation between changes in intakes in dietary fiber and grain products and changes in weight and development of obesity among middle aged women." American Journal of Clinical Nutrition 78:920-7.

Jacobson, M.F. and J. Hurley. 2002. *Restaurant Confidential*. Workman Publishing, New York, NY.

McArdle, W.D., F.I. Katch, and V.L. Katch. 1991. *Exercise Physiology: Energy, Nutrition, and Human Performance,* Third ed. Lea and Febiger, Malvern, PA.

Millward, D.J. 1998. "Metabolic demands for amino acids and the human dietary requirement." *Journal of Nutrition* 2563S-2576S.

Morris, K., et al. 1999. "Glycemic index, cardiovascular disease, and obesity." *Nutrition Reviews* 57:273-276.

Murray, M.T. and J. Beutler. 1996. *Understanding Fats and Oils*. Progressive Health Publishing, Encinitas, CA.

Nelson, J.K., et al. 1994. *Mayo Clinic Diet Manual: A Handbook of Nutrition Practices,* Seventh ed. Mosby, St. Louis, MO.

Netzer, C.T. 2003. *The Complete Book of Food Counts*. Dell Publishing, New York, NY.

Nicholl, C.G., J.M. Polak, and S.R. Bloom. 1985. "The hormonal regulation of food intake, digestion, and absorption." *Annual Review of Nutrition* 5:213-239.

Nobels, F., et al. 1989. "Weight reduction with a high protein, low carbohydrate, caloric restricted diet: Effects on blood pressure, glucose, and insulin levels." *Netherlands Journal of Medicine* 35:295-302.

Pieke., B., et al. 2000. "Treatment of hypertriglyceridemia by two diets rich either in unsaturated fatty acids or in carbohydrates: Effects on lipoprotein subclasses, lipolytic enzymes, lipid transfer proteins, insulin, and leptin. *International Journal of Obesity* 24:1286-1296.

Pilkis, S.J., et al. 1988. "Hormonal regulation of hepatic gluconeogenesis and glycolysis." *Annual Review of Biochemistry* 57:755-783.

Rabast, U., J. Schonborn, and H. Kasper. 1979. "Dietetic treatment of obesity with low- and high-carbohydrate diets: comparative studies and clinical results." *International Journal of Obesity* 3(3):201-11.

Reed, W.D., et al. 1984. "The effects of insulin and glucagons on ketone-body turnover." *Biochemistry* 221:439-444.

Reeds, P.J. and T.W. Hutchens. 1994. "Protein requirements: From nitrogen balance to functional impact." *Journal of Nutrition* 1754S-1963-S.

Richter, E.A., T. Ploug, and H. Galbo. 1985. "Increased muscle glucose uptake after exercise." *Diabetes* 34:1041-1048.

Scriver, C.R., et al. 1985. "Normal plasma amino acid values in adults: The influence of some common physiological variables." *Metabolism* 34:868-873.

Sears, B. and B. Lawren. 1995. *Enter the Zone*. Harper Collins, New York, NY.

Sims, E.A. 1974. "Studies in human hyperphagia." *Treatment and Management of Obesity.* New York, Harper and Row.

Souba, W.W., R.J. Smith, and D.W. Wilmore. 1985. "Glutamine Metabolism by the intestinal tract." *Journal of Parenteral Enteral Nutrition* 9:608-617.

Stewart, K.J., A.C. Bacher, K. Turner, et al. 2005. "Exercise and Risk Factors Associated with Metabolic Syndrome in Older Adults." *American Journal of Preventative Medicine* 28(1):9-18.

Stordy, B.J., et al. 1977. "Weight gain, thermic effects of glucose and resting metabolic rate during recovery from anorexia nervosa." *American Journal of Clinical Nutrition* 30:138.

The Life Application Study Bible NIV translation.1991. Tyndale and Zondervan. Tyndale House Publishers, Wheaton, IL.

Thorne, A. and J. Wahren. 1989. "Diet-induced thermogenesis in well-trained subjects." *Clinical Physiology* 0:295-305.

Traxinger, R.R. and S. Marshall. 1989. "Role of amino acids in modulating glucose-induced desensitization of the glucose transport system." *Journal of Biological Chemistry* 264:20910-20916.

Underwood, A. and J. Adler. Jan. 17, 2005 "Diet and genes." *Newsweek* 40-8.

Weinstein, A.R., H.P. Sesso, I.M. Lee., et al. 2004. "Relationship of physical activity versus body mass index with type II diabetes in women." *Journal of the American Medical Association* 292;10:1188-9.

Wessel, T.R., C.B. Arant, M.B. Olson, et al. 2004. "Relationship of physical fitness versus body mass index with coronary artery disease and cardiovascular events in women." *Journal of the American Medical Association* 292;10:1179-87.

Westphal, S.A., M.C. Gannon, and F.Q. Nutrall. 1990. "Metabolic response to glucose ingested with various amounts of protein." *American Journal of Clinical Nutrition* 62:267-272.

Whitney, E.N. and S.R. Rolfes. 1996. *Understanding Nutrition,* Seventh ed. West Publishing Company, St. Paul, MN.

Woods, S.C., et al. 1998. "Signals that regulate food intake and energy homeostasis." *Science* 280:1378-1383.

Wolfe, B.M. 1995. "Potential role of raising dietary protein intake for reducing risk of atherosclerosis." *Canadian Journal of Cardiology* 11:127G-131G.

Yamada, T., et al. 1995. *Textbook of Gastroenterology,* Second ed. J.B. Lippincott Company, Philadelphia, PA.

Young, D.B., et al. 1984. "Effects of sodium intake on steady-state potassium excretion." *American Journal of Physiology* 246:F772-F778.

Young, V.R. and J.S. Marchini. 1990. "Mechanisms and nutritional significance of metabolic responses to altered intakes of protein and amino acids, with reference to nutritional adaption in humans." *American Journal of Clinical Nutrition* 51:270-289.